The Complete
Quick & Hearty
Diabetic Cookbook
Second Edition

More than 200 Fast, Low-Fat Recipes with Old-Fashioned Good Taste

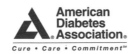

American Diabetes Association®

Cure • Care • Commitment℠

Managing Editor, Book Publishing, Abe Ogden; *Acquisitions Editor, Consumer Books,* Robert Anthony; *Editor,* Laurie Guffey; *Production Manager,* Melissa Sprott; *Composition & Cover Design,* American Diabetes Association; *Printer,* Data Reproductions Corporation.

Printed in the United States of America
3 5 7 9 10 8 6 4 2

The suggestions and information contained in this publication are generally consistent with the *Clinical Practice Recommendations* and other policies of the American Diabetes Association, but they do not represent the policy or position of the Association or any of its boards or committees. Reasonable steps have been taken to ensure the accuracy of the information presented. However, the American Diabetes Association cannot ensure the safety or efficacy of any product or service described in this publication. Individuals are advised to consult a physician or other appropriate health care professional before undertaking any diet or exercise program or taking any medication referred to in this publication. Professionals must use and apply their own professional judgment, experience, and training and should not rely solely on the information contained in this publication before prescribing any diet, exercise, or medication. The American Diabetes Association—its officers, directors, employees, volunteers, and members—assumes no responsibility or liability for personal or other injury, loss, or damage that may result from the suggestions or information in this publication.

⊗ The paper in this publication meets the requirements of the ANSI Standard Z39.48-1992 (permanence of paper).

ADA titles may be purchased for business or promotional use or for special sales. To purchase more than 50 copies of this book at a discount, or for custom editions of this book with your logo, contact Lee Romano Sequeira, Special Sales & Promotions, at the address below, or at LRomano@diabetes.org or 703-299-2046.

For all other inquiries, please call 1-800-DIABETES.

American Diabetes Association
1701 North Beauregard Street
Alexandria, Virginia 22311

Library of Congress Cataloging-in-Publication Data
The complete quick & hearty diabetic cookbook / American Diabetes Association. -- 2nd ed.
    p. cm.
 Originally published in 1998.
 Includes bibliographical references and index.
 ISBN 978-1-58040-285-9 (alk. paper)
 1. Diabetes--Diet therapy--Recipes. I. American Diabetes Association. II. Title: Complete quick and hearty diabetic cookbook.

RC662.C63 2007
641.5'6314--dc22

2007007460

Contents

Appetizers   1

Dressings & Sauces   23

Salads   35

Soups & Stews   59

Pasta   81

Poultry   99

Beef, Pork, & Lamb   131

Seafood   155

Vegetables   181

Rice & Potatoes   203

Breads & Muffins   215

Breakfasts   229

Desserts   241

Index   275

Appetizers

Baked Scallops, 3

Broiled Shrimp with Garlic, 4

Cheesy Tortilla Wedges, 5

Cherry Tomatoes Stuffed with Crab, 6

Chicken Kabobs, 7

Chilled Shrimp, 8

Crab Cakes, 9

Crab-Filled Mushrooms, 10

Creamy Tarragon Dip, 11

Cucumber Paté, 12

Fresh Dill Dip, 13

Gruyere Apple Spread, 14

Guacamole, 15

Hot Artichoke Dip, 16

Hot Crab Dip, 17

Hummus, 18

Low-Fat Cream Cheese Dip, 19

Monterey Jack Cheese Quiche Squares, 20

Stuffed Shrimp, 21

Turkey Meatballs, 22

NUTRITION FACTS

4 Servings
Serving Size 3 oz

AMOUNT PER SERVING

Exchanges
1 Lean Meat

Calories	70
Calories from Fat	8
Total Fat	1 g
Saturated Fat	0 g
Cholesterol	29 mg
Sodium	152 mg
with added salt	216 mg
Total Carbohydrate	2 g
Dietary Fiber	1 g
Sugars	1 g
Protein	13 g

Baked Scallops

Spear these scallops with fancy toothpicks or serve them on a bed of butter lettuce as a prelude to a pasta dish. Remember not to overcook scallops; they will become chewy instead of tender.

12 oz fresh bay or sea scallops
1/2 tsp salt (optional)
1 1/2 tsp pickling spices
1/2 cup cider vinegar

1/4 cup water
1 Tbsp finely chopped onion
1 head butter lettuce

1. Preheat the oven to 350 degrees. Wash the scallops in cool water and cut any scallops that are too big in half.
2. Spread scallops out in a large baking dish (be careful not to overlap them). Combine the spices, cider vinegar, water, and onion together in a small bowl and pour the mixture over the scallops.
3. Cover the baking dish and bake for 7 minutes. Remove from the oven and allow the scallops to cool in the refrigerator (leave them in the cooking liquid).
4. Just before serving, place lettuce leaves on individual plates or a platter and serve.

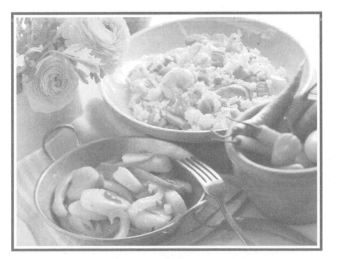

Broiled Shrimp with Garlic

*You can prepare this fast appetizer as guests are walking in,
or serve it as a main course over rice.
Make sure you buy two pounds of unshelled shrimp.*

2 lb large shrimp, unshelled

1/3 cup olive oil

1 Tbsp lemon juice

1/4 cup chopped scallions

1 Tbsp chopped garlic

2 tsp fresh ground pepper

1 large lemon, sliced

4 Tbsp chopped fresh parsley

1. Set the oven to broil. Shell uncooked shrimp, but do not remove the tails. With a small knife, split the shrimp down the back and remove the vein. Wash the shrimp with cool water and pat dry with paper towels.

2. In a medium skillet, over medium heat, heat the olive oil. Add the lemon juice, scallions, garlic, and fresh pepper. Heat the mixture for 3 minutes. Set aside.

3. Arrange the shrimp in a baking dish and pour the olive oil mixture over the shrimp. Broil the shrimp 4 to 5 inches from the heat for 2 minutes per side just until the shrimp turns bright pink. Transfer the shrimp to a platter and garnish with lemon slices and parsley. Pour the juices from the pan over the shrimp.

NUTRITION FACTS

12 Servings
Serving Size 2 1/2 oz

AMOUNT PER SERVING

Exchanges
2 Lean Meat

Calories	115	
Calories from Fat	60	
Total Fat	7	g
Saturated Fat	1	g
Cholesterol	120	mg
Sodium	139	mg
Total Carbohydrate	1	g
Dietary Fiber	0	g
Sugars	0	g
Protein	13	g

Cheesy Tortilla Wedges

These wedges are like nachos, except they are much lower in fat and calories.

6 large corn tortillas
1 cup shredded fat-free cheddar cheese

7 Tbsp shredded reduced-fat Monterey Jack cheese
1/2 cup green chiles
1/2 cup sliced pitted black olives

1. Preheat the oven to 400 degrees. Place tortillas on cookie sheets and bake 5 to 7 minutes or until edges start to curl.
2. Turn tortillas over; top with the two cheeses, chiles, and olives, spreading to the edge. Bake an additional 3 minutes or until cheese melts.
3. Cut each tortilla into 6 wedges and arrange on a platter. Top with Guacamole (optional; see recipe, page 15) and serve.

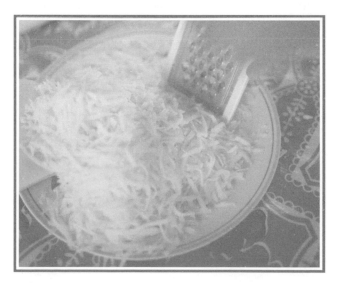

Cherry Tomatoes Stuffed with Crab

These bite-sized morsels with a fresh crabmeat filling are easy to make and fun to eat.

36 large cherry tomatoes
1 tsp salt
1/4 cup low-fat cottage cheese
1 1/2 tsp minced onion
1/2 tsp prepared horseradish
1 1/2 tsp fresh lemon juice
1/8 tsp garlic powder

1/2 lb cooked fresh crabmeat, flaked
1/4 cup minced celery
1 Tbsp finely chopped green bell pepper
Parsley leaves

1. Cut the tops off the tomatoes with a small knife and remove the pulp with a small spoon (use demitasse spoons, if you have them, or a small spoon with a pointed tip).
2. Sprinkle the insides of each tomato with salt. Invert the tomatoes on paper towels and let them drain while you prepare the filling.
3. Place the cottage cheese in a food processor or blender and process until smooth (about 2 minutes). Add the onion, horseradish, lemon juice, and garlic powder and process 1 more minute. Stir in the crabmeat, celery, and green pepper.
4. Stuff each tomato with some of the crabmeat filling. Arrange on a serving platter and refrigerate for at least 1 hour before serving. Garnish each tomato with a parsley leaf.

NUTRITION FACTS
12 Servings
Serving Size
  3 cherry tomatoes

AMOUNT PER SERVING

Exchanges
1 Vegetable

Calories   35
   Calories from Fat   4
Total Fat   0 g
   Saturated Fat   0 g
Cholesterol   8 mg
Sodium   275 mg
Total Carbohydrate   3 g
   Dietary Fiber   1 g
   Sugars   2 g
Protein   5 g

Chicken Kabobs

These are great served in the summer with roasted corn and squash.

1 lb boneless, skinless chicken breast

3 Tbsp lite soy sauce

1 1-inch cube of fresh ginger root, finely chopped

3 Tbsp olive oil

3 Tbsp dry vermouth

1 large clove garlic, finely chopped

12 watercress sprigs

2 large lemons, cut into wedges

1. Cut chicken into 1-inch cubes and place in a shallow bowl. Combine the soy sauce, ginger root, oil, vermouth, and garlic and pour over the chicken. Cover the chicken and let marinate overnight.

2. Thread the chicken onto 12 metal or wooden skewers (remember to soak the wooden skewers in water before using). Grill or broil 6 inches from the heat source for 8 minutes, turning frequently.

3. Arrange skewers on a platter and garnish with watercress and lemon wedges. Serve hot with additional soy sauce, if desired.

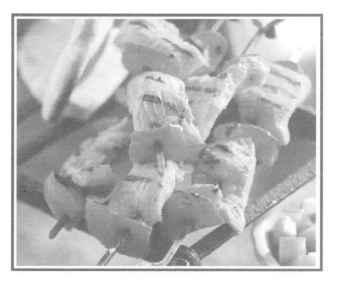

Chilled Shrimp

Your guests will appreciate this nicely chilled shrimp in a pretty combination of red onion, parsley, and lemon. Make sure you buy 5 pounds of unshelled shrimp.

5 lb jumbo shrimp, unshelled
1/4 cup plus 2 Tbsp olive oil
4 medium lemons, thinly sliced
3 Tbsp minced garlic

3 medium red onions, thinly sliced
1/2 cup minced parsley
Parsley sprigs

1. Peel and devein shrimp, leaving tails intact.

2. Preheat the oven to 400 degrees. Arrange the shrimp on a baking sheet and brush with 2 Tbsp olive oil. Bake the shrimp for 3 minutes or until they turn bright pink.

3. Place the lemon slices in a large bowl. Add the remaining 1/4 cup of olive oil, garlic, onions, and minced parsley. Add the shrimp and toss vigorously to coat. Cover and let marinate, refrigerated, for 6 to 8 hours.

4. Just before serving, arrange the shrimp on a serving platter. Garnish with parsley sprigs and some of the red onions and lemons from the bowl.

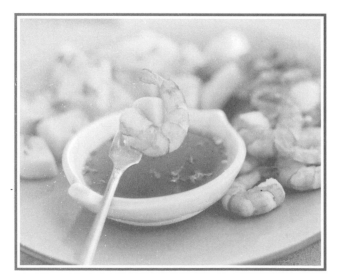

NUTRITION FACTS
20 Servings
Serving Size 2 1/2 oz

AMOUNT PER SERVING

Exchanges
2 Lean Meat

Calories	94	
Calories from Fat	26	
Total Fat	3	g
Saturated Fat	0	g
Cholesterol	151	mg
Sodium	174	mg
Total Carbohydrate	0	g
Dietary Fiber	0	g
Sugars	0	g
Protein	16	g

Crab Cakes

*Golden brown and full of flavor, crab cakes are great
the night of your party, and you can use the leftovers to make
crab cake sandwiches the next day.*

1 lb cooked fresh crabmeat
2 Tbsp finely minced parsley
2 Tbsp fat-free milk
1/2 tsp cayenne pepper
1/2 tsp dry mustard
2 Tbsp finely chopped onion
2 Tbsp finely chopped celery

1/2 cup egg substitute
1/2 tsp freshly ground pepper
8 slices low-calorie bread, crusts
  removed and finely crumbled
10 unsalted crackers, crushed into
  crumbs

1. In a medium bowl, combine all the ingredients except the cracker crumbs. Coat a baking sheet with nonstick cooking spray; set aside.

2. Shape the crabmeat mixture into 12 patties about 3 inches in diameter and 1/2 inch thick. Coat each patty with the cracker crumbs and place on the baking dish. Refrigerate the crab cakes 1 hour before baking. Preheat the oven to 400 degrees.

3. Bake the crab cakes at 400 degrees for 8 minutes or until golden brown. Transfer to a serving platter and serve hot.

Crab-Filled Mushrooms

~

This is a very versatile filling you can also stuff into cherry tomatoes, zucchini, or yellow squash "boats" (cut 2-inch pieces of squash and scoop out the middles).

20 large fresh mushroom caps
6 oz canned crabmeat, rinsed, drained, and flaked
2 Tbsp chopped fresh parsley
2 Tbsp finely chopped green onion

2 Tbsp Homemade Seasoned Bread Crumbs (see recipe, page 223)
Fresh ground pepper
1/4 cup chopped pimiento
3 Tbsp olive oil

1. Clean mushrooms by dusting off any dirt on the cap with a mushroom brush or paper towel; remove stems.
2. In a small mixing bowl, combine the crabmeat, parsley, green onion, bread crumbs, and pepper.
3. Place the mushroom caps in a 13 × 9 × 2-inch baking dish crown side down. Stuff some of the crabmeat filling into each cap. Place a little pimiento on top of the filling. Cover and refrigerate overnight.
4. Drizzle olive oil over each cap. Bake at 350 degrees for 15 to 17 minutes. Transfer to a serving platter and serve hot.

NUTRITION FACTS

10 Servings
Serving Size 2 mushrooms

AMOUNT PER SERVING

Exchanges
1 Vegetable
1 Fat

Calories	66
Calories from Fat	41
Total Fat	5 g
Saturated Fat	1 g
Cholesterol	15 mg
Sodium	53 mg
Total Carbohydrate	3 g
Dietary Fiber	1 g
Sugars	1 g
Protein	4 g

Creamy Tarragon Dip

This dip resembles a French boursin; it's especially good if you refrigerate it for 1 to 2 hours before serving to let the flavors blend.

2 tsp fresh or 1 tsp dried tarragon
2 tsp minced scallions
2 tsp minced parsley
1 cup low-fat cottage cheese

2 Tbsp tarragon vinegar
1 oz low-fat cream cheese, softened
1 tsp Dijon mustard

Combine all the ingredients in a food processor and process until smooth. Refrigerate until guests arrive; serve with raw vegetables or crackers.

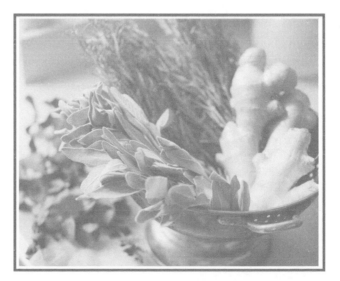

Cucumber Paté

You might want to make this tasty paté the day before your party, so it can solidify in the refrigerator overnight.

1 large cucumber, peeled, seeded, and quartered

1 small green bell pepper, seeded and quartered

3 stalks celery, quartered

1 medium onion, quartered

1 cup low-fat cottage cheese

1/2 cup low-fat mayonnaise

1 package unflavored gelatin

1/4 cup boiling water

1/4 cup cold water

1. Spray a 5-cup mold or a 1 1/2–quart mixing bowl with nonstick cooking spray.
2. In a food processor, coarsely chop the cucumber, green pepper, celery, and onion. Remove the vegetables from the food processor and set aside. Combine the cottage cheese and mayonnaise in the food processor and blend until smooth.
3. In a medium bowl, dissolve the gelatin in boiling water; slowly stir in the cold water. Add the chopped vegetables and cottage cheese mixture and mix thoroughly.
4. Pour the mixture into the prepared mold and refrigerate overnight or until firm. To serve, carefully invert mold onto serving plate and remove the mold. Surround the paté with assorted crackers and serve.

NUTRITION FACTS
12 Servings
Serving Size 1/2 cup

AMOUNT PER SERVING

Exchanges
1 Vegetable
1 Fat

Calories	61
Calories from Fat	32
Total Fat	4 g
Saturated Fat	1 g
Cholesterol	6 mg
Sodium	146 mg
Total Carbohydrate	4 g
Dietary Fiber	1 g
Sugars	3 g
Protein	4 g

Fresh Dill Dip

The fresh dill really adds great flavor to this dip.

1 cup plain fat-free yogurt
1/2 tsp salt (optional)
1/4 tsp fresh ground pepper
1/4 cup minced parsley

2 Tbsp chopped fresh chives
1 Tbsp chopped fresh dill
1 Tbsp apple cider vinegar

In a small bowl, combine all the ingredients. Chill for 2 to 4 hours. Serve with fresh cut vegetables.

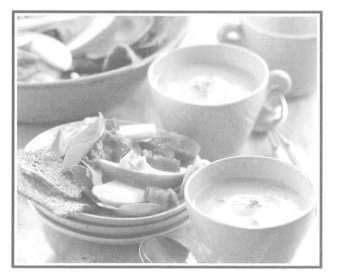

Gruyere Apple Spread

We've left the heavy ingredients out of this rich spread, tasty with crackers or fresh, raw vegetables.

4 oz fat-free cream cheese, softened
1/2 cup low-fat cottage cheese
4 oz Gruyere cheese
1/4 tsp dry mustard

1/2 cup shredded apple (unpeeled)
2 Tbsp finely chopped pecans
2 tsp minced chives

1. Place the cheeses in a food processor and blend until smooth. Add the mustard and blend for 30 seconds.

2. Transfer the mixture to a serving bowl and fold in the apple and pecans. Sprinkle the dip with chives.

3. Cover and refrigerate the mixture for 1 to 2 hours. Serve chilled with crackers or stuff into celery stalks.

NUTRITION FACTS
10 Servings
Serving Size 2 Tbsp

AMOUNT PER SERVING

Exchanges
1 Lean Meat

Calories	57	
Calories from Fat	27	
Total Fat	3	g
Saturated Fat	1	g
Cholesterol	8	mg
Sodium	145	mg
Total Carbohydrate	2	g
Dietary Fiber	0	g
Sugars	1	g
Protein	5	g

NUTRITION FACTS

8 Servings
Serving Size 1/4 cup

AMOUNT PER SERVING

Exchanges
1 Vegetable
2 1/2 Fat

Calories	132
Calories from Fat	102
Total Fat	11 g
Saturated Fat	2 g
Cholesterol	0 mg
Sodium	11 mg
with added salt	146 mg
Total Carbohydrate	9 g
Dietary Fiber	5 g
Sugars	3 g
Protein	2 g

Guacamole

There's a secret to selecting perfectly ripe avocados: look for slightly blackened ones that give just a little when you press on their skins.

2 large ripe avocados, peeled, pits removed, and mashed

1/2 chopped onion

2 medium jalapeño chile peppers, seeded and chopped

2 Tbsp minced fresh parsley

2 Tbsp fresh lime juice

1/8 tsp fresh ground pepper

2 medium tomatoes, finely chopped

1 medium garlic clove, minced

1 Tbsp olive oil

1/2 tsp salt (optional)

In a large mixing bowl, combine all ingredients, blending well. Cover and refrigerate for at least 1 to 2 hours.

Hot Artichoke Dip

Fresh Parmesan cheese gives this dip a special flavor.

2 15-oz cans artichoke hearts,
  packed in water, drained
2 cloves garlic
2 Tbsp olive oil
1/3 cup fresh lemon juice
1/4 tsp hot pepper sauce

1/4 cup grated fresh Parmesan
  cheese
2 cups dried bread crumbs
1/2 tsp dried oregano
1/2 tsp dried basil
1/4 tsp paprika
1/4 tsp dried thyme

1. Preheat the oven to 350 degrees. In a blender or food processor, puree the first five ingredients for 30 seconds. Pour the puree into a large bowl; stir in the cheese, bread crumbs, and herbs. Transfer the mixture to a 1-quart baking dish.
2. Cover the dip and bake for 15 minutes or until lightly golden brown. Serve warm with crackers or bread.

NUTRITION FACTS
32 Servings
Serving Size 2 Tbsp

AMOUNT PER SERVING

Exchanges
1/2 Starch

Calories	41	
Calories from Fat	13	
Total Fat	1	g
Saturated Fat	0	g
Cholesterol	1	mg
Sodium	128	mg
Total Carbohydrate	6	g
Dietary Fiber	1	g
Sugars	1	g
Protein	2	g

NUTRITION FACTS

6 Servings
Serving Size 1/3 cup

AMOUNT PER SERVING

Exchanges
2 Very Lean Meat

Calories	70	
Calories from Fat	3	
Total Fat	0	g
Saturated Fat	0	g
Cholesterol	29	mg
Sodium	364	mg
Total Carbohydrate	3	g
Dietary Fiber	0	g
Sugars	2	g
Protein	11	g

Hot Crab Dip

This dip is delicious with chunks of thick, crusty sourdough bread.

7 oz canned or cooked fresh crabmeat, rinsed, drained, and flaked
1/2 tsp horseradish
1/4 tsp paprika

8 oz fat-free cream cheese, softened
1 Tbsp fat-free milk
2 Tbsp fresh lemon juice

1. Preheat the oven to 350 degrees. In a medium bowl, combine all ingredients, blending thoroughly.
2. Spoon mixture into a small casserole dish and bake for 15 minutes until mixture bubbles. Serve hot with bread or crackers.

Hummus

❬⟋⟍❭

This recipe for this traditional Middle Eastern dip contains a lot less fat than other recipes; it's delicious with raw carrots or pita bread.

1 15-oz can chickpeas, drained
  (reserve a little liquid)
3–6 garlic cloves
Juice of 1 lemon

Juice of 1 lime
1 tsp olive oil
1 tsp ground cumin

Combine all ingredients in a blender or food processor until smooth, adding chickpea liquid if necessary to blend. Refrigerate. Serve with crunchy vegetables, crackers, or pita bread.

NUTRITION FACTS
12 Servings
Serving Size 2 Tbsp

AMOUNT PER SERVING

Exchanges
1/2 Starch

Calories	49	
Calories from Fat	9	
Total Fat	1	g
Saturated Fat	0	g
Cholesterol	0	mg
Sodium	39	mg
Total Carbohydrate	8	g
Dietary Fiber	1	g
Sugars	2	g
Protein	2	g

Low-Fat Cream Cheese Dip

You can use this basic recipe in several different ways. As written, it's perfect when you need plain cream cheese to serve with bagels. Add minced herbs such as parsley or chives (or pureed berries) to make flavored cream cheese. The frosting recipe with fructose added (see page 263) is delicious on baked goods!

1 1/3 cups plain fat-free yogurt, strained overnight in cheesecloth over a bowl set in the refrigerator

3 cups fat-free ricotta cheese
2 cups low-fat cottage cheese

Combine all the ingredients in a food processor; process until smooth. Place in a covered container and refrigerate until ready to use (this cream cheese can be refrigerated for up to 1 week).

Monterey Jack Cheese Quiche Squares

The green chiles add a special flavor to this delicious quiche.

3/4 cup egg substitute

1 cup plus 2 Tbsp low-fat cottage cheese

1/4 cup plus 2 Tbsp flour

3/4 tsp baking powder

1 cup shredded reduced-fat Monterey Jack cheese

1/2 cup diced green chiles

2 Tbsp diced red bell pepper

Parsley sprigs

1. Preheat the oven to 350 degrees. Beat egg substitute and cottage cheese together in a medium bowl for 2 minutes until smooth.

2. Add the flour and baking powder and beat until smooth. Stir in the cheese, green chiles, and red pepper.

3. Coat a square 9-inch pan with nonstick cooking spray and pour in egg mixture. Bake for 30 to 35 minutes until firm.

4. Remove the quiche from the oven and allow to cool for 10 minutes (it will be easier to cut). Cut into 12 squares and transfer to a platter, garnish with parsley sprigs, and serve.

NUTRITION FACTS

12 Servings
Serving Size 1 square

AMOUNT PER SERVING

Exchanges
1/2 Carbohydrate
1 Lean Meat

Calories	69
Calories from Fat	22
Total Fat	2 g
Saturated Fat	1 g
Cholesterol	10 mg
Sodium	218 mg
Total Carbohydrate	5 g
Dietary Fiber	0 g
Sugars	1 g
Protein	7 g

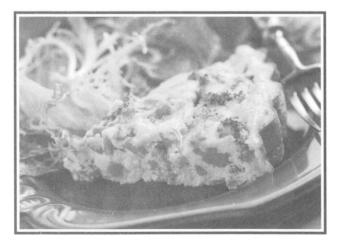

Stuffed Shrimp

This recipe calls for butterflied shrimp. Your fish market will do this for you if you wish—or simply make a deeper knife cut and flatten the jumbo shrimp after peeling and deveining.

1 cup dried bread crumbs

2 Tbsp dry vermouth

1 Tbsp grated fresh Parmesan cheese

1 1/2 tsp minced fresh parsley

1/4 cup olive oil

1 Tbsp paprika

1 garlic clove, minced

8 jumbo shrimp, shelled, deveined, and butterflied

1 medium lemon, sliced into wedges

1. Preheat the oven to 400 degrees. Coat a large baking dish with nonstick cooking spray or lightly grease with olive oil or margarine.
2. In a small bowl, combine the bread crumbs, vermouth, Parmesan cheese, parsley, olive oil, paprika, and garlic. Mix thoroughly.
3. In the baking dish, arrange the shrimp, cut side up. Mound the filling equally among all the shrimp, pressing to compact filling.
4. Bake the shrimp for 7 to 8 minutes or until the tops are golden brown.
5. Transfer the shrimp to a platter and garnish with lemon wedges.

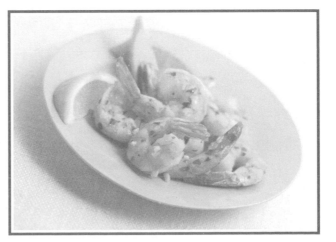

Turkey Meatballs

This is a healthy version of a great Italian appetizer.

1 lb ground turkey
1/4 cup low-sodium chicken broth
1/4 tsp allspice
1 slice low-calorie bread, finely
  crumbled
1/4 cup egg substitute

4 tsp fresh lemon juice
1/4 tsp ground nutmeg
2 Tbsp finely chopped green onion
1/2 tsp grated lemon peel
1 1/4 cups low-fat, low-sodium
  marinara sauce

1. Preheat the oven to 400 degrees. Coat a shallow baking dish with non-stick cooking spray and set aside.

2. Combine all the ingredients except the marinara sauce in a medium bowl, mixing thoroughly. Form the mixture into tiny meatballs, about 1 tsp each.

3. Place the meatballs on the baking sheet and bake for 10 minutes or until well browned all over. Remove from the oven and arrange on a serving platter. Spear each turkey meatball with a fancy toothpick. Serve with 1 Tbsp of marinara sauce per serving.

NUTRITION FACTS
20 Servings
Serving Size 2–3 meatballs

AMOUNT PER SERVING

Exchanges
1 Lean Meat

Calories	47	
Calories from Fat	21	
Total Fat	2	g
Saturated Fat	1	g
Cholesterol	12	mg
Sodium	27	mg
Total Carbohydrate	2	g
Dietary Fiber	0	g
Sugars	1	g
Protein	5	g

Dressings & Sauces

Basic Barbecue Sauce, 25

Basic Vinaigrette, 26

Creamy Herb Dressing, 27

Dill Dressing, 28

French Dressing, 29

Ginger-Soy Dressing, 30

Marinara Sauce, 31

Mock Hollandaise, 32

Parmesan Dressing, 33

Tangy Marinade, 34

Basic Barbecue Sauce

This homemade version has none of the chemicals found in many bottled brands. You need to make up a fresh batch when you need it, or make ahead and store it in the freezer, though.

1 Tbsp olive oil	Fresh ground pepper
1 medium onion, chopped	1 Tbsp white vinegar
1 1/4 cups tomato sauce	1/4 tsp dry mustard
1 bay leaf	1/4 tsp hot pepper sauce
1/4 tsp curry powder	1 Tbsp chopped parsley

1. In a medium saucepan, heat the oil and sauté the onion until tender, about 5 minutes.

2. Add the remaining ingredients and simmer for 20 minutes.

3. Discard the bay leaf and transfer the sauce to a container.

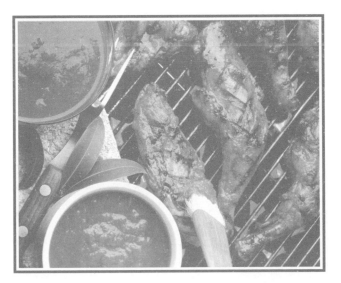

Basic Vinaigrette

Spice up this basic dressing with chopped, fresh herbs such as basil or dill.

3/4 cup olive oil

3 Tbsp fresh lemon juice

1 garlic clove, minced

2 Tbsp white wine vinegar

2 tsp Dijon mustard

1 tsp minced fresh parsley

Dash salt and pepper

Combine all ingredients in a blender or food processor. Process until well blended. Refrigerate until ready to use.

NUTRITION FACTS

24 Servings
Serving Size 1 Tbsp

AMOUNT PER SERVING

Exchanges
1 1/2 Fat

Calories	61	
Calories from Fat	61	
Total Fat	7	g
Saturated Fat	1	g
Cholesterol	0	mg
Sodium	11	mg
Total Carbohydrate	0	g
Dietary Fiber	0	g
Sugars	0	g
Protein	0	g

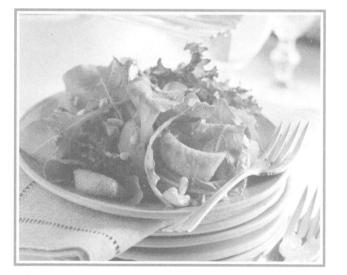

NUTRITION FACTS

24 Servings
Serving Size 1 Tbsp

AMOUNT PER SERVING

Exchanges
Free Food*

Calories	11	
Calories from Fat	2	
Total Fat	0	g
Saturated Fat	0	g
Cholesterol	43	mg
Sodium	43	mg
with added salt	64	mg
Total Carbohydrate	1	g
Dietary Fiber	0	g
Sugars	1	g
Protein	2	g

*Remember that only 2 Tbsp
or less is a Free Food!

Creamy Herb Dressing

*Use this low-fat, low-calorie creamy dressing over salad greens
or as a dip for vegetables.*

1/2 cup plain fat-free yogurt   1/2 tsp dried thyme
1 cup low-fat cottage cheese   1/4 tsp dried marjoram
1 1/2 tsp fresh lemon juice   1/4 tsp dried oregano
1 medium carrot, peeled and grated   1/4 tsp dried basil
2 tsp grated onion   1/4 tsp salt (optional)

1. In a food processor, combine the yogurt, cottage cheese, and lemon juice;
   process until smooth. Pour into a small mixing bowl.
2. Add the remaining ingredients and mix well. Cover and refrigerate for
   1 to 2 hours before serving.

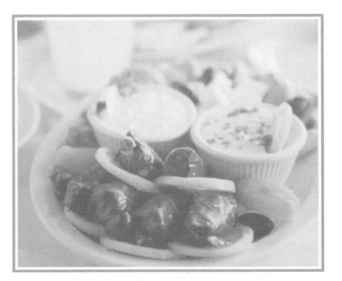

Dill Dressing

Try this dressing with fresh grilled salmon or swordfish.

1/2 cup plain fat-free yogurt

2 Tbsp low-fat mayonnaise

2 tsp grated onion

1 garlic clove, minced

1/4 cup fat-free milk

1 tsp dried dill or 2 tsp chopped
  fresh dill

1/4 tsp dried oregano

Fresh ground pepper

Combine all ingredients in a food processor or blender and process until smooth. Pour into a container, cover, and refrigerate for 1 to 2 hours before serving.

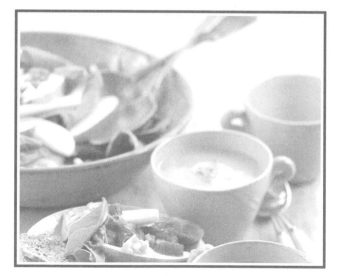

French Dressing

This dressing makes a special impression on dinner guests, with its pleasing aroma and pretty color.

1/2 cup olive oil
1/4 cup malt vinegar
1 tsp salt (optional)

Dash lemon pepper
Dash paprika
1/4 tsp dry mustard

Combine all ingredients in a blender or food processor. Process until well blended. Refrigerate until ready to use.

Ginger-Soy Dressing

This dressing can double as a marinade for chicken, turkey, or fish.

1/2 cup lite soy sauce

2 Tbsp sesame oil

2 Tbsp rice vinegar

1 Tbsp grated fresh ginger

1 Tbsp dry sherry

1 tsp granulated sugar substitute

Combine all ingredients in a small jar, cover tightly, and shake vigorously until well blended. Keep covered and refrigerated until ready to serve. Shake again before serving.

NUTRITION FACTS

16 Servings
Serving Size 1 Tbsp

AMOUNT PER SERVING

Exchanges
1/2 Fat

Calories	20	
Calories from Fat	15	
Total Fat	2	g
Saturated Fat	0	g
Cholesterol	0	mg
Sodium	300	mg
Total Carbohydrate	1	g
Dietary Fiber	0	g
Sugars	1	g
Protein	0	g

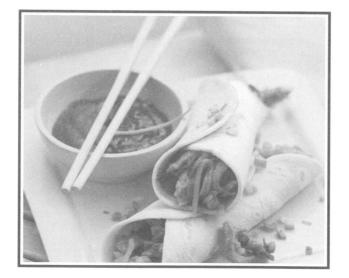

Marinara Sauce

Keep a batch on hand in the freezer. The taste complements shrimp or pasta and is a great dipping sauce for baked chicken fingers.

24 oz tomato puree
1 green bell pepper, chopped
1 red bell pepper, chopped
1/2 cup minced onion

1 tsp dried oregano
1/2 lb mushrooms, sliced
1 tsp dried basil
1/2 tsp garlic powder

In a large saucepan over medium heat, combine all ingredients, mixing thoroughly. Let simmer 40 to 50 minutes, allowing flavors to blend.

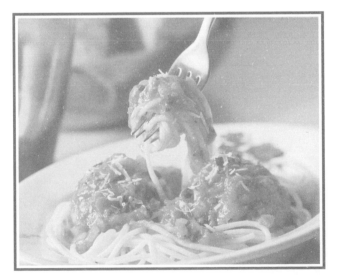

Mock Hollandaise

Use over any fresh, lightly steamed vegetable.

1/2 cup low-fat mayonnaise   1 Tbsp lemon juice
3 Tbsp water   Fresh ground white pepper

1. In a small saucepan, combine all ingredients. Whisk until smooth.

2. Simmer mixture over low heat, stirring constantly, for 3 to 4 minutes until heated through.

NUTRITION FACTS
4 Servings
Serving Size 2 Tbsp

AMOUNT PER SERVING

Exchanges
2 Fat

Calories	101	
Calories from Fat	83	
Total Fat	9	g
Saturated Fat	1	g
Cholesterol	12	mg
Sodium	221	mg
Total Carbohydrate	2	g
Dietary Fiber	0	g
Sugars	1	g
Protein	0	g

NUTRITION FACTS

16 Servings
Serving Size 1 Tbsp

AMOUNT PER SERVING

Exchanges
1 1/2 Fat

Calories	65
Calories from Fat	63
Total Fat	7 g
Saturated Fat	1 g
Cholesterol	1 mg
Sodium	18 mg
with added salt	26 mg
Total Carbohydrate	1 g
Dietary Fiber	0 g
Sugars	1 g
Protein	0 g

Parmesan Dressing

*This dressing also tastes good with cooked broccoli,
string beans, or asparagus.*

1/2 cup white wine vinegar
3 Tbsp Parmesan cheese
1 garlic clove, minced
Dash salt (optional)

1/2 cup olive oil
1 tsp dried basil
Fresh ground pepper

Place all ingredients in a jar and cover. Shake vigorously and refrigerate until ready to use.

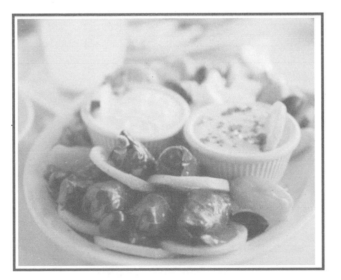

Tangy Marinade

This recipe is great for marinating beef or pork before grilling. Store extra portions in the freezer.

1 cup unsweetened pineapple juice
1 garlic clove, minced
1/3 cup lite soy sauce

1 tsp ground ginger
1/3 cup low-calorie Italian
   salad dressing

In a shallow dish, combine all ingredients, mixing thoroughly. Keep refrigerated until ready to use.

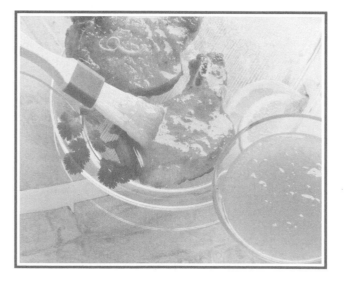

Exchanges
1/2 Starch

Calories	44
Calories from Fat	0
Total Fat	0 g
Saturated Fat	0 g
Cholesterol	0 mg
Sodium	870 mg
Total Carbohydrate	9 g
Dietary Fiber	0 g
Sugars	9 g
Protein	1 g

Salads

Black Bean Salad, 37

California Seafood Salad, 38

Chinese Chicken Salad, 39

Couscous Salad, 40

Crab and Rice Salad, 41

Fresh Seafood Pasta Salad, 42

Greek Potato Salad, 43

Green Bean, Walnut, and Feta Salad, 44

Italian Potato Salad, 45

Lentil Salad, 46

Lobster Salad, 47

Mediterranean Chicken Salad, 48

Overnight Coleslaw, 49

Pasta Salad–Stuffed Tomatoes, 50

Shanghai Salad, 51

Shrimp and Pasta Salad, 52

Shrimp and Radicchio Salad, 53

Tabbouleh Salad, 54

Tortellini and Feta Cheese Salad, 55

Wild Rice Salad, 56

Zucchini and Carrot Salad, 57

Black Bean Salad

Try this spicy salad with grilled chicken or pork.

3 cups cooked black beans
2 tomatoes, chopped
2 red bell peppers, finely chopped
1 cup yellow corn
3 garlic cloves, minced
1 jalapeño pepper, minced

1/4 cup fresh lime juice
2 Tbsp red wine vinegar
1 Tbsp cumin
1 Tbsp olive oil
2 Tbsp chopped fresh cilantro
(optional)

Combine all ingredients in a bowl and refrigerate for several hours to blend the flavors. Serve.

California Seafood Salad

Try using pieces of crab or lobster instead of, or in addition to, the shrimp and scallops.

1/4 lb fresh green beans, cut into
   1-inch pieces
1 Tbsp olive oil
1 lb fresh scallops
1 lb uncooked fresh shrimp,
   shelled and deveined
1/2 cup low-fat sour cream
2 Tbsp low-fat mayonnaise

2 Tbsp fat-free milk
1 Tbsp chopped fresh dill
2 Tbsp chopped fresh parsley
2 Tbsp fresh lime juice
1 head romaine lettuce
1 large tomato, cut into wedges
1 lemon, cut into wedges

1. To prepare the salad, steam the green beans for 3 to 4 minutes until cooked, but slightly crunchy. Set aside. In a large skillet, heat the olive oil.

2. Add the scallops and shrimp and sauté over medium heat for 4 to 5 minutes until the seafood is cooked (the shrimp turn pink and the scallops are no longer translucent). Set aside to cool while you prepare the dressing.

3. Combine all the dressing ingredients together in a small bowl. Add the dressing to the seafood and mix well. Add the green beans and toss again.

4. To assemble, place lettuce leaves on individual plates or one platter. Place seafood salad in a mound on top of the lettuce. Surround the salad with tomato and lemon wedges.

NUTRITION FACTS

8 Servings
Serving Size 4 oz

AMOUNT PER SERVING

Exchanges
1 Vegetable
2 Lean Meat

Calories	143	
Calories from Fat	45	
Total Fat	5	g
Saturated Fat	1	g
Cholesterol	87	mg
Sodium	226	mg
Total Carbohydrate	7	g
Dietary Fiber	2	g
Sugars	4	g
Protein	18	g

Chinese Chicken Salad

*This is a crunchy salad, loaded with sweet pineapple
and crisp water chestnuts.*

2 cups cooked chicken, diced
1 cup finely chopped celery
1/4 cup crushed unsweetened pineapple, drained
2 Tbsp finely diced pimiento
2 8-oz cans water chestnuts, drained
and chopped

2 scallions, chopped
1/3 cup low-fat mayonnaise
1 Tbsp lite soy sauce
1 tsp lemon juice
8 large tomatoes, hollowed

1. In a large bowl, combine the chicken, celery, pineapple, pimiento, water chestnuts, and scallions.

2. In a separate bowl, combine the mayonnaise, soy sauce, and lemon juice. Mix well. Add the dressing to the salad and toss. Cover and refrigerate for 2 to 3 hours.

3. For each serving, place a small scoop of chicken salad into a hollowed-out tomato. You may also stuff the chicken salad into celery stalks or serve on bread.

Couscous Salad

Couscous, also known as Moroccan pasta, is very simple to prepare. Place dry couscous in a heat-proof bowl, pour double the amount of boiling water or broth over it, and let it sit for 5 to 10 minutes until all the water is absorbed.

1 cup couscous, rehydrated (see above)

1/4 cup finely chopped red or yellow bell pepper

1/4 cup chopped carrots

1/4 cup finely chopped celery

2 Tbsp minced Italian parsley

1 Tbsp olive oil

4 Tbsp rice vinegar

2 garlic cloves, minced

3 Tbsp finely minced scallions

Fresh ground pepper

1. Combine the couscous, vegetables, and minced parsley together in a large bowl.
2. Combine the remaining ingredients in a blender or food processor and process for 1 minute. Pour over the couscous and vegetables, toss well, and serve.

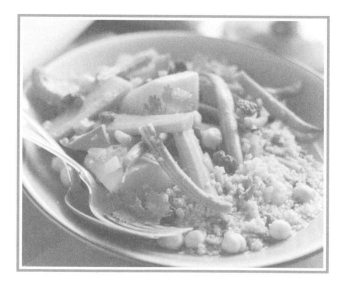

Exchanges
2 Starch
1/2 Fat

Calories	191	
Calories from Fat	42	
Total Fat	5	g
Saturated Fat	1	g
Cholesterol	0	mg
Sodium	20	mg
Total Carbohydrate	32	g
Dietary Fiber	2	g
Sugars	4	g
Protein	5	g

Crab and Rice Salad

Brown rice gives this salad a great nutty taste.

1 cup uncooked brown rice
5 oz cooked fresh crabmeat, flaked
1 large tomato, diced
1/4 cup chopped green bell pepper
3 Tbsp chopped fresh parsley
2 Tbsp red onion

1/2 cup plain fat-free yogurt
1 1/2 Tbsp lemon juice
1/4 tsp salt (optional)
Fresh ground pepper
1 head butter lettuce
1 large tomato, cut into wedges

1. In a medium saucepan, boil 2 1/2 cups of water. Slowly add 1 cup uncooked brown rice. Cover and reduce the heat to low. Cook the rice for 45 to 50 minutes until tender. Do not continually stir the rice (this will cause it to become gummy). Just check occasionally.

2. In a large salad bowl, combine all the ingredients except the lettuce and tomato wedges. Just before serving, line plates with the lettuce and spoon salad on top of the lettuce. Garnish with tomato wedges.

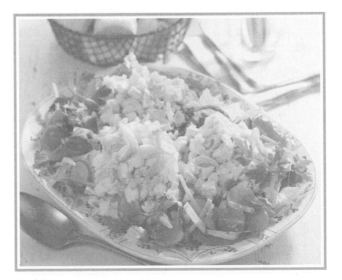

Fresh Seafood Pasta Salad

~

This is a delicious medley of fresh fish, pasta, and vegetables.

3/4 cup broccoli florets
22 oz uncooked fresh shrimp, shelled and deveined
1 lb cooked small pasta shells
2 medium carrots, peeled and diced
1/2 medium red onion, diced
4 Tbsp chopped cilantro
1 each red, yellow, and green bell pepper, julienned
8 large cherry tomatoes, halved

4 medium celery stalks, diced
4 scallions, chopped
2 Tbsp minced garlic
12 large pitted black olives
1/2 lb cooked sea scallops
1/2 lb cooked fresh crabmeat, flaked
1/2 cup olive oil
1/3 cup red wine vinegar
Fresh ground pepper

1. To a large pot of boiling water, add the broccoli florets and then turn off the heat. After 1 minute, rinse the broccoli under cold running water to stop the cooking process, then drain. (This method of blanching helps the broccoli to retain its bright green color and crispness.)
2. Boil the shrimp until it just turns pink. Combine the pasta and vegetables in a large salad bowl. Add the cooked seafood and toss with the pasta and vegetables.
3. Combine the oil, vinegar, and pepper. Pour the dressing over the salad and refrigerate for several hours before serving.

NUTRITION FACTS
12 Servings
Serving Size 3/4 cup

AMOUNT PER SERVING

Exchanges
1 Starch
1 Vegetable
1 Medium-Fat Meat
1 Fat

Calories	226	
Calories from Fat	97	
Total Fat	11	g
Saturated Fat	2	g
Cholesterol	90	mg
Sodium	242	mg
Total Carbohydrate	17	g
Dietary Fiber	2	g
Sugars	5	g
Protein	16	g

NUTRITION FACTS
10 Servings
Serving Size 1/2 cup

AMOUNT PER SERVING

Exchanges
1 Starch
1 Vegetable
1 1/2 Fat

Calories	177	
Calories from Fat	74	
Total Fat	8	g
Saturated Fat	1	g
Cholesterol	0	mg
Sodium	237	mg
Total Carbohydrate	25	g
Dietary Fiber	4	g
Sugars	4	g
Protein	3	g

Greek Potato Salad

You'll love this unique potato salad, served warm, with its authentic flavor of Kalamata olives (Greek olives). Find them at your supermarket or a gourmet deli.

1/3 cup olive oil
4 garlic cloves, minced
2 lb red potatoes, cut into 1 1/2–inch pieces (leave the skin on if you wish)
6 medium carrots, peeled, halved lengthwise, and cut into 1 1/2-inch pieces

1 onion, chopped
16 oz artichoke hearts packed in water, drained and cut in half
1/2 cup Kalamata olives, pitted and halved
1/4 cup lemon juice
Dash salt and pepper

1. In a large skillet, heat the olive oil, add the garlic, and sauté for 30 seconds. Add the potatoes, carrots, and onion; cook over medium heat for 25 to 30 minutes until vegetables are just tender.

2. Add the artichoke hearts and cook for 3 to 5 minutes more. Remove from heat and stir in the olives and lemon juice. Season with salt and pepper. Transfer to a serving bowl and serve warm.

Green Bean, Walnut, and Feta Salad

Make sure to toast the walnuts—the roasted flavor really enhances this salad.

1/2 cup walnuts

1 1/2 lb fresh green beans, trimmed and halved

1 medium red onion, sliced into rings

1/2 cup peeled, seeded, and diced cucumber

1/3 cup crumbled fat-free feta cheese

1/4 cup olive oil

1/4 cup white wine vinegar

1/4 cup chopped fresh mint leaves

1 garlic clove, minced

1/2 tsp salt (optional)

1. Toast the walnuts by placing them in a small baking dish in a 350-degree oven for 5 to 10 minutes until lightly browned. Remove from the oven and set aside.
2. Steam the green beans about 4 to 5 minutes, or until desired degree of crispness.
3. In a salad bowl, combine the green beans with the walnuts, red onion rings, cucumber and feta cheese. Combine all the dressing ingredients together and toss with the vegetables. Chill 2 to 3 hours before serving.

NUTRITION FACTS
12 Servings
Serving Size 1/2 cup

AMOUNT PER SERVING

Exchanges
1 Vegetable
1 1/2 Fat

Calories	103	
Calories from Fat	71	
Total Fat	8	g
Saturated Fat	1	g
Cholesterol	0	mg
Sodium	100	mg
with added salt	197	mg
Total Carbohydrate	7	g
Dietary Fiber	2	g
Sugars	2	g
Protein	5	g

NUTRITION FACTS

6 Servings
Serving Size 1/2 cup

AMOUNT PER SERVING

Exchanges
1 Starch
1 Vegetable
1/2 Fat

Calories	122
Calories from Fat	42
Total Fat	5 g
Saturated Fat	1 g
Cholesterol	0 mg
Sodium	29 mg
Total Carbohydrate	19 g
Dietary Fiber	3 g
Sugars	1 g
Protein	2 g

Italian Potato Salad

The warm, earthy taste of balsamic vinegar gives this salad its punch. Leave the skins on the red potatoes for a rustic look.

24 new red potatoes, 3–4 oz each, washed and skins left on
3 celery stalks, chopped
1 red bell pepper, minced
1/4 cup chopped scallions

2 Tbsp olive oil
1 Tbsp balsamic vinegar
1/2 Tbsp red vinegar
1 tsp chopped fresh parsley
Fresh ground pepper

1. Boil the potatoes for 20 minutes in a large pot of boiling water. Drain and let cool for 30 minutes. Cut potatoes into large chunks and toss the potatoes with the celery, red pepper, and scallions.

2. Combine all the dressing ingredients and pour over the potato salad. Serve at room temperature.

Lentil Salad

The flavor of this filling salad improves with time, so you can leave the leftovers in the refrigerator for 2 to 3 days and serve it again!

1 lb dried lentils, washed (rinse with cold water in a colander)

3 cups water

2 Tbsp olive oil

2 tsp cumin

1 tsp minced fresh oregano

3 Tbsp fresh lemon juice

Fresh ground pepper

2 large green bell peppers, cored, seeded, and diced

2 large red bell peppers, cored, seeded, and diced

3 stalks celery, diced

1 red onion, minced

1. In a large saucepan over high heat, bring lentils and water to a boil. Reduce the heat to low, cover, and simmer for 35 to 45 minutes. Drain and set aside.

2. In a large bowl, mix together the oil, lemon juice, cumin, oregano, and pepper until well blended. Add the lentils and the prepared vegetables. Cover and refrigerate before serving.

Lobster Salad

Lobster is a special treat your guests will appreciate.

2 lb lobster in the shell
  or 1 lb lobster meat
3/4 lb small red potatoes
1/2 cup low-fat mayonnaise
3 Tbsp plain low-fat yogurt

1 Tbsp chopped tarragon
1/4 cup chopped scallions
Fresh ground pepper
1 small head romaine lettuce,
  washed and leaves separated

1. To prepare lobster in the shell, place the lobster in boiling water and boil until meat is tender, about 20 minutes. Cool the lobster, remove the meat from the shell, and cut into 1-inch cubes. Or buy lobster meat from the seafood department at the supermarket.

2. Wash, but do not peel, the potatoes. Boil the potatoes in water until just tender, about 15 to 20 minutes. Drain, cool, and quarter. In a bowl, combine the remaining dressing ingredients. In a separate bowl, combine the lobster and potatoes.

3. Add dressing to the lobster and potatoes and mix well. To serve, line plates with lettuce. Spoon lobster salad over the lettuce.

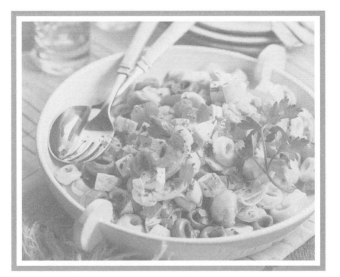

Mediterranean Chicken Salad

*Try adding crumbled fat-free feta cheese to this salad
to give it more of a Greek flair.*

8 oz boneless, skinless, cooked chicken breast

2 Tbsp olive oil

2 Tbsp balsamic vinegar

1/4 tsp dried basil

2 small garlic cloves, minced

Fresh ground pepper

1 cup cooked green beans, cut into 2-inch lengths

1/4 cup sliced black olives

3 cherry tomatoes, halved

Tomato wedges (optional)

1. Cut the cooked chicken into bite-sized chunks and set aside. In a medium bowl, whisk together the oil, vinegar, basil, garlic, and pepper. Add the chicken and toss with dressing.

2. Add the green beans, olives, and cherry tomatoes; toss well. Refrigerate for several hours. Garnish salad with tomato wedges and serve.

NUTRITION FACTS

3 Servings
Serving Size 1/3 recipe

AMOUNT PER SERVING

Exchanges
3 Very Lean Meat
2 Vegetable
2 Fat

Calories	244
Calories from Fat	116
Total Fat	13 g
Saturated Fat	2 g
Cholesterol	64 mg
Sodium	157 mg
Total Carbohydrate	7 g
Dietary Fiber	2 g
Sugars	3 g
Protein	25 g

Overnight Coleslaw

*This salad gets all its flavor from spices and apple juice
instead of high-fat mayonnaise.*

4 cups shredded cabbage (green or
   purple, or a mixture)
2 cups shredded carrots
3/4 cup sliced scallions
3/4 cup unsweetened apple juice
2/3 cup cider vinegar

1 1/2 tsp paprika
1 tsp mustard seeds
1/2 tsp garlic powder
1/2 tsp celery seeds
Fresh ground pepper
1 Tbsp dry mustard

1. Combine the cabbage, carrots, and scallions.
2. Combine the remaining ingredients in a blender and pour over the cabbage mixture. Toss to coat. Refrigerate overnight and serve chilled.

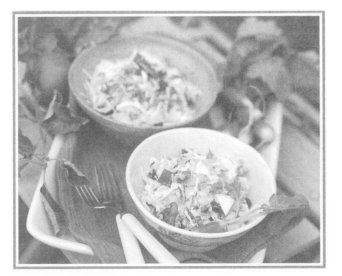

Pasta Salad–Stuffed Tomatoes

This is a lovely salad to serve for a light luncheon.

1 cup uncooked corkscrew macaroni

2 small carrots, sliced

2 scallions, chopped

1/4 cup chopped pimiento

1 cup cooked kidney beans

1/2 cup sliced celery

1/4 cup cooked peas

2 Tbsp chopped fresh parsley

1/4 cup low-calorie Italian salad dressing

2 Tbsp low-fat mayonnaise

1/4 tsp dried marjoram

Fresh ground pepper

4 medium tomatoes

1. Cook the corkscrew macaroni in boiling water until cooked, about 7 to 8 minutes; drain.

2. In a large mixing bowl, combine the macaroni with the remaining salad ingredients and toss well. Cover and chill 1 hour or more.

3. With the stem end down, cut each tomato into 6 wedges, cutting to, but not through, the base of the tomato. Spread wedges slightly apart and spoon pasta mixture into tomatoes. Chill until ready to serve.

NUTRITION FACTS

4 Servings
Serving Size 2/3 cup stuffing in 1 medium tomato

AMOUNT PER SERVING

Exchanges
2 Starch
1 Vegetable
1/2 Fat

Calories	207
Calories from Fat	34
Total Fat	4 g
Saturated Fat	1 g
Cholesterol	3 mg
Sodium	303 mg
Total Carbohydrate	37 g
Dietary Fiber	7 g
Sugars	9 g
Protein	8 g

Shanghai Salad

Use last night's leftover steak to create this warm Asian salad.

3 Tbsp canola oil
1 tsp grated ginger
1 garlic clove, minced
8 oz cooked lean flank steak, cut into 1-inch pieces
1 1/2 cups fresh snow peas, trimmed
1 8-oz can water chestnuts, drained and sliced
6 scallions, cut into 2-inch pieces
2 Tbsp dry sherry
1 Tbsp lite soy sauce
4 cups romaine lettuce, shredded

1. In a large skillet, heat the oil over medium-high heat. Sauté the ginger and garlic for 1 to 2 minutes.

2. Add the remaining ingredients except lettuce to the skillet and stir until heated through.

3. Arrange shredded lettuce on platter, spoon mixture over the bed of lettuce, and serve.

Shrimp and Pasta Salad

*Shells, shrimp, and a bit of Romano cheese make
this salad tasty and festive.*

1 lb uncooked shell macaroni
12 oz frozen baby shrimp
6 scallions, thinly sliced
3 small zucchini, sliced
10 cherry tomatoes, halved
1 Tbsp dried Italian seasoning

1 Tbsp minced fresh garlic
Fresh ground pepper
1 Tbsp Romano cheese
1/4 cup olive oil
1/3 cup red wine vinegar
1 small head butter lettuce

1. Cook the shell macaroni in boiling water for 6 to 7 minutes, adding the
   frozen shrimp after 4 minutes. Drain.

2. In a large bowl, combine the macaroni, shrimp, scallions, zucchini, and
   tomatoes. Sprinkle with Italian seasoning, garlic, pepper, and cheese
   and mix well.

3. Drizzle the olive oil and vinegar on top and toss until well coated; refrigerate until chilled. To serve, line a clear glass bowl with lettuce leaves
   and spoon mixture into the bowl.

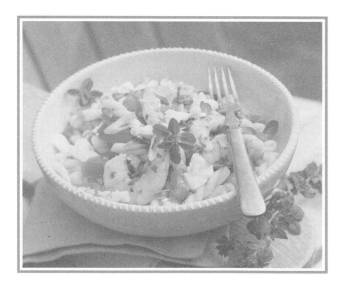

NUTRITION FACTS
8 Servings
Serving Size 1 cup

AMOUNT PER SERVING

Exchanges
3 Starch
1 Medium-Fat Meat

Calories	329
Calories from Fat	77
Total Fat	9 g
Saturated Fat	1 g
Cholesterol	72 mg
Sodium	105 mg
Total Carbohydrate	47 g
Dietary Fiber	3 g
Sugars	5 g
Protein	16 g

Shrimp and Radicchio Salad

Radicchio is a very beautiful lettuce—its burgundy color adds eye appeal to any salad.

1/4 cup olive oil
2 Tbsp red wine vinegar
3 medium garlic cloves, minced
1 medium shallot, minced
2 tsp Dijon mustard
1 tsp prepared horseradish

Fresh ground pepper
1/2 lb cooked bay shrimp
1 medium head Boston lettuce, shredded
1 medium head radicchio lettuce, shredded

1. In a medium bowl, combine all the dressing ingredients. Add the shrimp and toss well. Refrigerate for 30 minutes.
2. Just before serving, combine the lettuce and radicchio in a serving bowl. Place the shrimp mixture on top, toss, and serve.

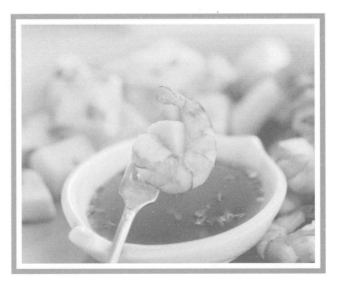

Tabbouleh Salad

You can find the bulgur wheat called for in this recipe in most supermarkets (look in the rice and pasta aisle).

1 cup bulgur wheat

2 cups boiling water

1 large tomato, chopped

1/2 cup minced fresh parsley

1/4 cup chopped scallions

1 Tbsp chopped fresh mint

1/4 cup fresh lemon juice

Dash salt and pepper

1 Tbsp olive oil

1 tsp ground cumin

1 small head butter lettuce

1 lemon, cut into wedges

1. In a small bowl, combine the wheat with the boiling water and let stand at room temperature for at least 1 hour, until the wheat has absorbed the water. The wheat will expand and should yield about 2 cups of rehydrated wheat.

2. Combine the tomato, parsley, scallions, and mint with the wheat and toss well. Combine the dressing ingredients and pour over the wheat salad. Cover and refrigerate overnight or for at least 2 to 3 hours.

3. To serve, place lettuce leaves on individual plates and spoon salad over lettuce leaves. Garnish with lemon wedges.

NUTRITION FACTS
8 Servings
Serving Size 1/2 cup

AMOUNT PER SERVING

Exchanges
1 Starch
1 Vegetable

Calories	104
Calories from Fat	19
Total Fat	2 g
Saturated Fat	0 g
Cholesterol	0 mg
Sodium	29 mg
Total Carbohydrate	20 g
Dietary Fiber	1 g
Sugars	7 g
Protein	3 g

NUTRITION FACTS

9 Servings
Serving Size 1/2 cup

AMOUNT PER SERVING

Exchanges
1 Starch
1 1/2 Fat

Calories	147
Calories from Fat	64
Total Fat	7 g
Saturated Fat	1 g
Cholesterol	3 mg
Sodium	286 mg
Total Carbohydrate	17 g
Dietary Fiber	2 g
Sugars	2 g
Protein	5 g

Tortellini and Feta Cheese Salad

A little bit of this salad goes a long way—it's packed with tortellini, walnuts, and feta cheese.

14 oz frozen reduced-fat cheese tortellini
2 Tbsp canola oil
2 Tbsp white wine vinegar
1/4 cup sliced scallions
1 garlic clove, finely minced
1 tsp dried basil

1 8-oz can water-packed artichoke hearts, drained and quartered
1/4 cup crumbled reduced-fat feta cheese
1/4 cup chopped black olives
1/4 cup chopped walnuts
1 large tomato, cut into 9 thin slices

1. Prepare the tortellini according to package directions (without adding salt); drain and cool.

2. In a small bowl, whisk together the oil and vinegar. Add scallions, garlic, basil, and dill; mix well.

3. Combine the remaining ingredients and pour the dressing on top. Refrigerate overnight or at least 2 to 3 hours. Garnish each serving with a tomato slice.

Wild Rice Salad

This salad has a slightly sweet flavor.

1 cup raw wild rice (rinsed)

4 cups cold water

1 cup mandarin oranges, packed in their own juice (drain and reserve 2 Tbsp of liquid)

1/2 cup chopped celery

1/4 cup minced red bell pepper

1 shallot, minced

1 tsp minced thyme

2 Tbsp raspberry vinegar

1 Tbsp olive oil

1. Place the rinsed, raw rice and the water in a saucepan. Bring to a boil, lower the heat, cover the pan, and cook for 45 to 50 minutes until the rice has absorbed the water. Set the rice aside to cool.

2. In a large bowl, combine the mandarin oranges, celery, red pepper, and shallot. In a small bowl, combine the reserved juice, thyme, vinegar, and oil. Add rice to the mandarin oranges and vegetables. Pour the dressing over the salad, toss, and serve.

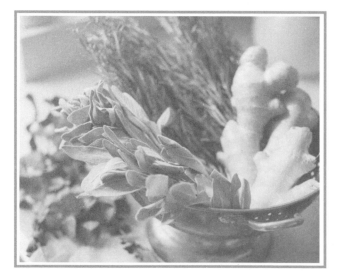

NUTRITION FACTS
4 Servings
Serving Size 1 cup

AMOUNT PER SERVING

Exchanges
2 1/2 Starch

Calories	205
Calories from Fat	36
Total Fat	4 g
Saturated Fat	1 g
Cholesterol	0 mg
Sodium	22 mg
Total Carbohydrate	38 g
Dietary Fiber	5 g
Sugars	7 g
Protein	6 g

NUTRITION FACTS

6 Servings
Serving Size 1/2 cup

AMOUNT PER SERVING

Exchanges
2 Vegetable
2 Fat

Calories	129	
Calories from Fat	95	
Total Fat	11	g
Saturated Fat	1	g
Cholesterol	0	mg
Sodium	155	mg
Total Carbohydrate	8	g
Dietary Fiber	3	g
Sugars	3	g
Protein	3	g

Zucchini and Carrot Salad

This salad features julienned ribbons of carrot, zucchini, and fennel in a delightful Dijon vinaigrette.

2 medium carrots, peeled and julienned
1 medium zucchini, julienned
1/2 medium fennel bulb, core removed and julienned
1 Tbsp fresh orange juice
2 Tbsp Dijon mustard
3 Tbsp olive oil

1 tsp white wine vinegar
1/2 tsp dried thyme
1 Tbsp finely minced parsley
Dash salt
Fresh ground pepper
1/4 cup chopped walnuts
1 medium head romaine lettuce, washed and leaves separated

1. Place julienned vegetables in a medium bowl and set aside.

2. Combine remaining ingredients, except walnuts and lettuce, and mix well. Pour dressing over vegetables and toss. Add walnuts and mix again. Refrigerate until ready to serve.

3. To serve, line a bowl or plates with lettuce leaves and spoon salad on top.

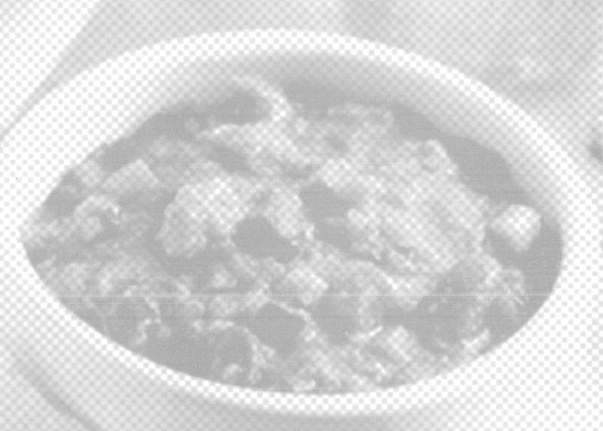

Soups & Stews

Chicken and Mushroom Soup, 61

Chicken Stew with Noodles, 62

Cream of Carrot Soup, 63

English Beef Stew, 64

French Onion Soup, 65

Fresh Fish Chowder, 66

Gazpacho, 67

Hearty Vegetable Soup, 68

Italian Minestrone, 69

Lentil Soup, 70

Mexican Tortilla Soup, 71

Mushroom and Barley Soup, 72

Old-Fashioned Vegetable Beef Stew, 73

Pasta Fagioli, 74

Potato Chowder, 75

Quick Manhattan Clam Chowder, 76

Quick Shrimp Gumbo, 77

Spanish Black Bean Soup, 78

Spicy Turkey Chili, 79

White Bean Soup, 80

Chicken and Mushroom Soup

Try serving this soup with fresh Buttermilk Biscuits (see recipe, page 219).

1 quart low-sodium chicken broth
1 Tbsp lite soy sauce
1 cup sliced mushrooms, stems removed

1 Tbsp finely chopped scallions
1 Tbsp dry sherry
1/2 lb boneless, skinless chicken breast, cubed

1. Simmer all ingredients except the chicken in a stockpot for 10 minutes.
2. Add the chicken cubes and simmer for 6 to 8 minutes more. Serve with additional soy sauce if desired (but be aware that this will raise the sodium level of the soup).

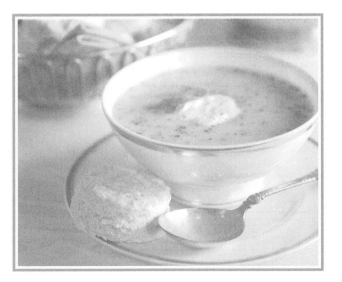

Chicken Stew with Noodles

Try using this stew to top rice or a baked potato.

1 Tbsp olive oil

1 onion, chopped

2 garlic cloves, minced

1 lb boneless, skinless chicken
   breast, cubed

2 Tbsp flour

3 cups low-sodium chicken broth

1 cup dry white wine

1 Tbsp chopped fresh thyme (or 1
   tsp dried)

1 lb cooked noodles, hot

1/2 cup minced parsley

1. In a large saucepan, heat the oil and sauté the onion and garlic for about 5 minutes. Add the chicken cubes and sauté until chicken is cooked (about 10 minutes).

2. Sprinkle the flour over the chicken. Add the chicken broth, wine, and thyme. Bring to a boil, then lower the heat and simmer for 30 minutes.

3. Toss together the noodles and the parsley. Pour the stew over the noodles and serve.

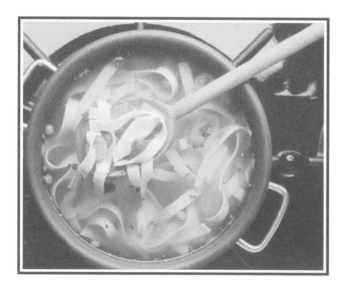

NUTRITION FACTS

8 Servings
Serving Size 1 cup stew and
   1/2 cup cooked noodles

AMOUNT PER SERVING

Exchanges
1 Starch
2 Lean Meat

Calories	191
Calories from Fat	42
Total Fat	5 g
Saturated Fat	1 g
Cholesterol	53 mg
Sodium	58 mg
Total Carbohydrate	19 g
Dietary Fiber	1 g
Sugars	3 g
Protein	17 g

Cream of Carrot Soup

This smooth, tasty soup is great to serve for special luncheons.

2 Tbsp low-sodium chicken broth
3 Tbsp finely chopped shallots or onions
2 Tbsp flour
1 cup fat-free milk, scalded and hot
1 tsp cinnamon
1 cup cooked, pureed carrots
1 cup low-sodium chicken broth
Fresh ground pepper

1. Heat the broth in a stockpot over medium heat. Add shallots and cook until they are limp. Sprinkle shallots with flour and cook 2 to 3 minutes.

2. Pour in the hot milk and cook until mixture thickens. Add remaining ingredients. Bring almost to a boil, stirring often. Add pepper to taste.

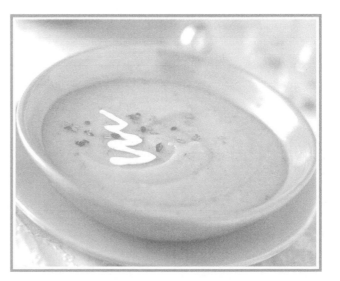

English Beef Stew

This stew has a slightly different flavor than Old-Fashioned Vegetable Beef Stew (see recipe, page 73), but is just as satisfying.

2 lb lean beef for stew, cut into large chunks
1 1/2 Tbsp flour
2 Tbsp canola oil
2 cups boiling water
2 tsp garlic powder
1 Tbsp Worcestershire sauce

Dash salt and pepper
1 large yellow onion, quartered
4 large carrots, peeled and quartered
3 medium potatoes, white or russet, cut into 1-inch cubes
1 cup canned stewed tomatoes

1. Roll the beef cubes in the flour. In a large saucepan over medium heat, heat the canola oil. Add the beef and sauté a few pieces of beef at a time. When all beef has been browned, add the boiling water to the pan.

2. Add the garlic powder, Worcestershire sauce, salt, and pepper. Lower the heat, cover, and let simmer for 2 to 2 1/2 hours or until the meat is very tender.

3. Add the onion, carrots, potatoes, and tomatoes. Let simmer about 30 minutes until all vegetables are just tender. Transfer to a serving bowl and serve.

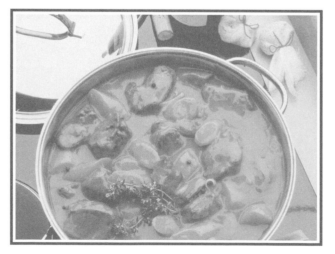

Exchanges
1 Starch
3 Lean Meat

Calories	256	
Calories from Fat	82	
Total Fat	9	g
Saturated Fat	2	g
Cholesterol	65	mg
Sodium	183	mg
Total Carbohydrate	20	g
Dietary Fiber	3	g
Sugars	7	g
Protein	23	g

French Onion Soup

This version of a very popular soup is altered slightly—the fat content is much lower, yet the authentic taste is all here.

5 tsp canola oil
1 lb yellow onions, thinly sliced
1 tsp brown sugar substitute
Fresh ground pepper (optional)
1 Tbsp unbleached flour
1 quart low-sodium, fat-free beef broth

1/3 cup vermouth
4 slices French bread, toasted (about 3/4-inch slices)
2 thin slices (1 1/3 oz) reduced-fat Swiss cheese, cut in half

1. In a large stockpot, heat the oil and sauté the onion for 15 minutes. Add the sugar substitute and pepper. Cook uncovered over low heat for 35 minutes, stirring occasionally, adding a little water if necessary. The onions will get very brown.

2. Add the flour and cook an additional 1 minute. Gradually add the beef broth and vermouth; cook over medium heat, stirring constantly until thickened and bubbly. Reduce the heat and simmer for 20 minutes.

3. Ladle the soup into 4 individual oven-safe soup bowls. Top each bowl with a slice of bread and half a slice of cheese. Place under the broiler for 2 to 3 minutes. Carefully remove from the oven and serve.

Fresh Fish Chowder

You can use almost any fish in this chowder—we've suggested halibut.

2 Tbsp olive oil

1 large garlic clove, minced

1 small onion, chopped

1 large green bell pepper, chopped

1 lb crushed tomatoes

1 Tbsp tomato paste

1/2 tsp dried basil

1/2 tsp dried oregano

1/4 cup dry red wine

Dash salt and pepper

1/2 cup uncooked white rice

1/2 lb fresh halibut, cubed

2 Tbsp chopped parsley

NUTRITION FACTS

6 Servings

Serving Size 1 cup

AMOUNT PER SERVING

Exchanges
1 Starch
1 Vegetable
1 Medium-Fat Meat

Calories	181
Calories from Fat	52
Total Fat	6 g
Saturated Fat	1 g
Cholesterol	12 mg
Sodium	72 mg
Total Carbohydrate	22 g
Dietary Fiber	2 g
Sugars	5 g
Protein	10 g

1. Heat the olive oil in a 3-quart saucepan. Add the garlic, onion, and green pepper; sauté for 10 minutes over low heat until vegetables are just tender.

2. Add the tomatoes, tomato paste, basil, oregano, wine, salt, and pepper. Let simmer for 15 minutes. Add the rice and continue to cook for 15 minutes.

3. Add the halibut and cook for about 5 to 7 minutes until fish is cooked through. Garnish stew with chopped parsley and serve.

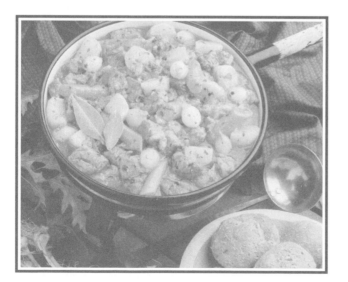

NUTRITION FACTS

4 Servings
Serving Size 1 1/2 cups

AMOUNT PER SERVING

Exchanges
1 Starch
1 Vegetable
1/2 Fat

Calories	136	
Calories from Fat	44	
Total Fat	5	g
Saturated Fat	1	g
Cholesterol	1	mg
Sodium	412	mg
Total Carbohydrate	20	g
Dietary Fiber	5	g
Sugars	14	g
Protein	6	g

Gazpacho

*Serve this cool, refreshing vegetable and tomato
broth on hot summer days.*

1 garlic clove, crushed
1 Tbsp olive oil
1 large onion, chopped
5 medium tomatoes, peeled
1 cup low-sodium chicken broth
2 Tbsp red wine vinegar
1 tsp hot pepper sauce

1/4 tsp paprika
1 large green or red bell pepper,
    chopped
1 cup peeled, seeded, and chopped
    cucumber
1/4 cup chopped scallions

1. Combine the garlic, oil, onion, and tomatoes in a food processor and
   process until smooth. Add the broth, vinegar, hot pepper sauce, and
   paprika; process again. Transfer the mixture to a large soup tureen or
   bowl.

2. Add the red or green pepper, cucumber, and scallions. Chill in the refrigerator overnight. Serve the soup in bowls or large wine glasses. Top with
   croutons if desired.

Hearty Vegetable Soup

Try this soup with fresh-baked Corn Muffins (see recipe, page 220).

1 1/2 quarts low-sodium chicken broth

1 28-oz can whole tomatoes, chopped and drained

1 cup chopped onion

1 cup diced potatoes

1 cup sliced carrots

1 cup yellow corn

1 cup frozen or fresh shelled peas

1 cup cooked kidney, black, or pinto beans (drained and rinsed, if canned)

2 tsp oregano

1 Tbsp minced fresh parsley

1 bay leaf

Fresh ground pepper

Combine all ingredients in a large stockpot. Bring to a boil. Reduce the heat and simmer for 1 hour until vegetables are just tender. Remove bay leaf before serving.

NUTRITION FACTS

8 Servings
Serving Size about 1 cup

AMOUNT PER SERVING

Exchanges
1 1/2 Starch
1 Vegetable

Calories	142	
Calories from Fat	17	
Total Fat	2	g
Saturated Fat	0	g
Cholesterol	1	mg
Sodium	314	mg
Total Carbohydrate	26	g
Dietary Fiber	6	g
Sugars	7	g
Protein	7	g

NUTRITION FACTS

8 Servings
Serving Size 1 cup

AMOUNT PER SERVING

Exchanges
1 Starch
1 Vegetable

Calories	116
Calories from Fat	25
Total Fat	3 g
Saturated Fat	0 g
Cholesterol	0 mg
Sodium	188 mg
Total Carbohydrate	19 g
Dietary Fiber	4 g
Sugars	5 g
Protein	5 g

Italian Minestrone

This soup is traditionally served with warm, crusty French bread.

1 Tbsp olive oil
1/2 cup sliced onion
4 cups low-sodium chicken broth
3/4 cup sliced carrot
1/2 cup sliced potato (with peel)
2 cups sliced cabbage or coarsely
 chopped spinach
1 cup sliced zucchini
1/2 cup cooked garbanzo beans
 (drained and rinsed, if canned)

1/2 cup cooked navy beans
 (drained and rinsed, if canned)
16 oz canned tomatoes, with liquid
1/2 cup sliced celery
2 tsp dried basil
1 tsp dried oregano
1/2 cup uncooked rotini or
 other shaped pasta
1 Tbsp minced fresh parsley

1. In a large stockpot over medium heat, sauté the onion in oil until onion is slightly browned. Add the chicken broth, carrot, and potatoes. Cover and cook over medium heat for 30 minutes.

2. Add remaining ingredients and cook for an additional 15 to 20 minutes until the pasta is cooked through.

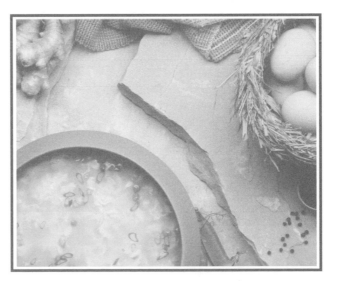

Lentil Soup

~

Cooking with lentils is a tasty and inexpensive way to include high-quality protein and complex carbohydrates in your diet—and they're easy to use because they don't require presoaking. This is a thick, hearty soup, perfect for a chilly day.

1 large onion, diced
1 large carrot, peeled and diced
2 stalks celery, diced
2 Tbsp olive oil
1 lb lentils

1 1/2 quarts low-sodium chicken or beef broth
2 medium russet or white potatoes, peeled and diced
1 tsp dried oregano
1 tsp dried thyme

1. In a stockpot or Dutch oven, sauté the onion, carrot, and celery in the olive oil for 10 minutes. Add the lentils, broth, and potatoes.

2. Continue to cook for 30 to 45 minutes, adding the oregano and thyme 15 minutes before serving. Soup will keep for 3 days in the refrigerator or can be frozen for 3 months.

NUTRITION FACTS
8 Servings
Serving Size 1 cup

AMOUNT PER SERVING

Exchanges
3 Starch
1/2 Fat

Calories	275	
Calories from Fat	48	
Total Fat	5	g
Saturated Fat	1	g
Cholesterol	1	mg
Sodium	75	mg
Total Carbohydrate	42	g
Dietary Fiber	13	g
Sugars	7	g
Protein	16	g

Mexican Tortilla Soup

Strips of tortillas lace this spicy, hearty soup.

2 tsp olive oil
1 onion, chopped
2 cloves garlic, minced
1 Tbsp chopped fresh cilantro
1 Tbsp cumin
1 tsp cayenne pepper
1 quart low-sodium chicken broth

1 15-oz can whole tomatoes, drained and coarsely chopped
1 medium zucchini, sliced
1 medium yellow squash, sliced
1 cup yellow corn
6 corn tortillas
1/2 cup shredded low-fat cheese (optional)

1. In a large saucepan, heat the oil and sauté the onion and garlic for 5 minutes.
2. Add the cilantro, cumin, and cayenne pepper; sauté for 3 more minutes. Add remaining ingredients except the tortillas and optional cheese. Bring to a boil; cover and let simmer for 30 minutes.
3. Cut each tortilla into about 10 strips. Place the strips on a cookie sheet and bake for 5 to 6 minutes at 350 degrees until slightly browned and toasted. Remove from the oven.
4. To serve the soup, place strips of tortilla into each bowl. Ladle the soup on top of the tortilla strips. Top with cheese if desired.

Mushroom and Barley Soup

Barley adds fiber and a rich flavor to soup.

1/2 cup barley

6 cups water

1 large carrot, diced

2 cups diced celery

2 bay leaves

1/4 cup minced fresh parsley

1 tsp dried thyme

1 medium onion, diced

2 Tbsp olive oil

1/2 lb mushrooms, sliced

1 garlic clove, minced

2 Tbsp lite soy sauce

2 Tbsp fresh lemon juice

Fresh ground pepper

1. Place barley and water in a 2-quart saucepan; bring to a boil. Reduce heat and let simmer; add carrot, celery, bay leaves, parsley, and thyme.

2. Return to a boil, reduce the heat, cover, and let simmer for 1 hour. When the barley has been cooking about 45 minutes, use a small skillet to sauté the onion in the olive oil for about 5 minutes.

3. Add the mushrooms and sauté until tender. Add the mushroom mixture to the barley, along with the remaining ingredients. Continue to simmer for 10 more minutes.

NUTRITION FACTS

6 Servings
Serving Size 1 cup

AMOUNT PER SERVING

Exchanges
1 1/2 Starch
1/2 Fat

Calories	140
Calories from Fat	45
Total Fat	5 g
Saturated Fat	1 g
Cholesterol	0 mg
Sodium	262 mg
Total Carbohydrate	22 g
Dietary Fiber	5 g
Sugars	5 g
Protein	3 g

NUTRITION FACTS

8 Servings
Serving Size 1 cup

AMOUNT PER SERVING

Exchanges
1 Starch
1 Vegetable
1 Lean Meat
1/2 Fat

Calories	193
Calories from Fat	64
Total Fat	7 g
Saturated Fat	2 g
Cholesterol	33 mg
Sodium	250 mg
Total Carbohydrate	20 g
Dietary Fiber	4 g
Sugars	7 g
Protein	14 g

Old-Fashioned Vegetable Beef Stew

*Loaded with chunky vegetables, this stew will
warm you up on a cold day!*

1 lb lean beef for stew, cut into
  1-inch cubes
2 Tbsp olive oil
1 medium onion, diced
2 garlic cloves, crushed
1 28-oz can tomatoes, slightly
  crushed
2 cups low sodium beef broth
2 large carrots, peeled and cut into
  1/4-inch round slices

1/2 lb mushrooms, sliced
1/2 lb green beans, cut into
  2-inch pieces
4 celery stalks, sliced diagonally
Fresh black pepper
Dash cayenne pepper
Dash hot pepper sauce
2 medium russet or white potatoes,
  peeled and cut into 1-inch cubes

1. In a large saucepan over medium heat, lightly brown the meat in the
   olive oil. Add the onion, garlic, tomatoes, and beef broth; bring to a boil.

2. Reduce to a simmer; add carrots, mushrooms, green beans, and celery.
   Season the soup with pepper, cayenne pepper, and hot pepper sauce.
   Cover and simmer for 45 minutes to 1 hour.

3. Add the potatoes and cook until just tender, adding water if necessary.
   Serve hot.

Pasta Fagioli

This hearty Italian soup freezes well, so you'll get several meals out of this recipe.

1 Tbsp olive oil
1 large onion, chopped
3 cloves garlic, crushed
2 medium carrots, sliced
2 medium zucchini, sliced
2 tsp basil
2 tsp oregano

1 32-oz can unsalted tomatoes with liquid
1 32-oz can white cannellini or navy beans, drained and rinsed
1 lb uncooked rigatoni or shell macaroni

1. Heat the oil in a large saucepan and sauté the onions and garlic for 5 minutes.

2. Add the carrots, zucchini, basil, oregano, tomatoes with their liquid, and the beans. Cook until the vegetables are just tender, about 15 to 17 minutes.

3. In a separate saucepot, cook the pasta according to package directions (without adding salt). Add the pasta to the soup and mix thoroughly. Serve warm with crusty bread.

NUTRITION FACTS

12 Servings
Serving Size 3/4–1 cup

AMOUNT PER SERVING

Exchanges
3 Starch
1 Vegetable

Calories	263
Calories from Fat	19
Total Fat	2 g
Saturated Fat	0 g
Cholesterol	0 mg
Sodium	115 mg
Total Carbohydrate	51 g
Dietary Fiber	4 g
Sugars	10 g
Protein	11 g

Potato Chowder

This is a creamy, low-fat version of a potato lover's favorite.

2 tsp olive oil
3/4 cup chopped onion
1/2 cup diced celery
1 bay leaf
1 clove garlic, minced
1/4 cup flour
1/4 cup evaporated fat-free milk
2 cups fat-free milk
3 1/2 cups low-sodium chicken broth

1 1/2 lb potatoes, peeled and cut into 2-inch cubes
1 tsp salt (optional)
1 tsp dried basil
1/4 tsp dried thyme
1/4 tsp nutmeg
1/4 tsp celery seeds
Fresh ground pepper
1 Tbsp cider vinegar
1 Tbsp minced parsley

1. In a large saucepan, heat the oil. Add the onion, celery, and bay leaf; cook over medium heat for 5 minutes, stirring occasionally.

2. Add garlic and slowly add the flour; mix well. Slowly add the evaporated milk, fat-free milk, and chicken broth. Bring to a boil, stirring constantly.

3. Add the potatoes, salt, basil, thyme, nutmeg, celery seeds, and pepper. Reduce the heat and let simmer, uncovered, for 25 to 30 minutes or until potatoes are just tender, stirring frequently.

4. Add the vinegar and discard the bay leaf. Remove 3 cups of the mixture and place in a food processor; puree. Add the mixture back to the stockpot and mix thoroughly. Sprinkle with parsley and serve.

Quick Manhattan Clam Chowder

Try serving this chunky chowder with hot sourdough bread.

3 medium carrots, peeled and coarsely chopped

3 large white or russet potatoes, peeled and coarsely chopped

4 celery stalks, coarsely chopped

2 1/2 cups minced clams, drained

2 cups canned tomatoes, slightly crushed

1 Tbsp imitation bacon bits (optional)

1/2 tsp dried thyme or 1 tsp minced fresh thyme

Dash salt and pepper

Add all the ingredients to a large stockpot. Cover and let simmer for 1 to 2 hours. Serve hot.

NUTRITION FACTS

8 Servings
Serving Size about 1 cup

AMOUNT PER SERVING

Exchanges
1 Lean Meat
1 1/2 Starch

Calories	161	
Calories from Fat	11	
Total Fat	1	g
Saturated Fat	0	g
Cholesterol	33	mg
Sodium	218	mg
with bacon bits	233	mg
Total Carbohydrate	23	g
Dietary Fiber	3	g
Sugars	7	g
Protein	15	g

NUTRITION FACTS

4 Servings
Serving Size 3 oz shrimp with
sauce and 1/4 cup rice

AMOUNT PER SERVING

Exchanges
1 Starch
1 Vegetable
1 Lean Meat

Calories	182
Calories from Fat	14
Total Fat	2 g
Saturated Fat	0 g
Cholesterol	167 mg
Sodium	396 mg
Total Carbohydrate	21 g
Dietary Fiber	2 g
Sugars	6 g
Protein	21 g

Quick Shrimp Gumbo

Serve this spicy gumbo with a fresh spinach salad and warm rolls.

2 cups canned tomatoes, undrained
1/4 cup chopped green bell pepper
1 medium onion, chopped
1 cup uncooked white rice
1/2 cup low-sodium chicken broth

1 medium garlic clove, minced
Dash hot pepper sauce
Fresh ground pepper
12 oz precooked jumbo shrimp

1. Place all the ingredients except the shrimp in a large stockpot and bring to a boil. Reduce the heat, cover, and let simmer for 25 to 30 minutes.

2. Add the shrimp, cover, and simmer for 5 to 10 minutes or until shrimp is thoroughly heated. Serve hot.

Spanish Black Bean Soup

*The combination of red wine and black beans
gives this soup its robust flavor.*

2 tsp chicken broth

1 tsp olive oil

3 garlic cloves, minced

1 yellow onion, minced

1 tsp minced fresh oregano

1 tsp cumin

1 tsp chili powder or 1/2 tsp cayenne pepper

1 red bell pepper, chopped

1 carrot, coarsely chopped

3 cups cooked black beans

1 1/2 cups low-sodium chicken
broth

1/2 cup dry red wine

1. In a large pot, heat the chicken broth and olive oil. Add the garlic and onions and sauté for 3 minutes. Add the oregano, cumin, and chili powder;
stir for another minute. Add the red pepper and carrot.

2. Puree 1 1/2 cups of the black beans in a blender or food processor. Add
the pureed beans, remaining 1 1/2 cups whole black beans, chicken
broth, and red wine to the stockpot. Simmer 1 hour. Taste before serving; add additional spices if you like.

NUTRITION FACTS

6 Servings
Serving Size 1 cup

AMOUNT PER SERVING

Exchanges
2 Starch

Calories	155
Calories from Fat	15
Total Fat	2 g
Saturated Fat	0 g
Cholesterol	0 mg
Sodium	29 mg
Total Carbohydrate	26 g
Dietary Fiber	6 g
Sugars	6 g
Protein	9 g

Spicy Turkey Chili

This chili tastes great with fresh-baked Corn Muffins
(see recipe, page 220).

(see recipe, page 220).

NUTRITION FACTS

6 Servings
Serving Size 1 cup

AMOUNT PER SERVING

Exchanges
1 1/2 Starch
2 Lean Meat

Calories	220	
Calories from Fat	32	
Total Fat	4	g
Saturated Fat	1	g
Cholesterol	51	mg
Sodium	175	mg
Total Carbohydrate	23	g
Dietary Fiber	5	g
Sugars	5	g
Protein	25	g

2 onions, chopped
2 garlic cloves, minced
1/2 cup chopped green bell pepper
1 Tbsp olive oil
1 lb lean ground turkey breast meat
2 cups kidney or pinto beans

2 cups canned tomatoes with liquid
1 cup low-sodium chicken broth
2 Tbsp chili powder
2 tsp cumin
Fresh ground pepper

1. In a large saucepan, sauté the onion, garlic, and green pepper in the oil for 10 minutes. Add the turkey and sauté until the turkey is cooked, about 5 to 10 minutes. Drain any fat away.

2. Add the remaining ingredients, bring to a boil, lower the heat, and simmer uncovered for 30 minutes. Add additional chili powder if you like your chili extra spicy.

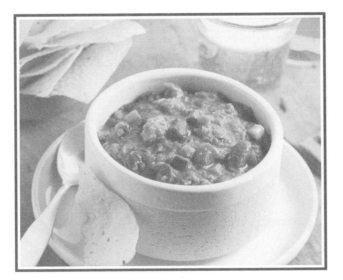

White Bean Soup

Use any variety of white bean for this scrumptious soup.

1/4 cup chopped onion
1 garlic clove, minced
2 Tbsp olive oil
1/2 lb dried great northern, white navy, or cannellini beans
2 quarts water

2 bay leaves
1 tsp dried basil
Dash salt and pepper
2 medium scallions, chopped
2 Tbsp minced fresh parsley

1. In a large saucepan, sauté the onion and garlic in the oil for 5 minutes. Add the beans, water, bay leaves, and basil; stir well. Bring mixture to a boil, reduce the heat, cover, and let simmer.

2. Continue to cook the soup for 2 hours or until beans are tender. Add water (if necessary), salt, and pepper; mix well.

3. In a blender or food processor, puree the mixture. Return the soup back to the saucepan and serve hot. Garnish with scallions and parsley.

NUTRITION FACTS
6 Servings
Serving Size 1 cup

AMOUNT PER SERVING

Exchanges
1 1/2 Starch
1/2 Fat

Calories	157	
Calories from Fat	43	
Total Fat	5	g
Saturated Fat	1	g
Cholesterol	0	mg
Sodium	28	mg
Total Carbohydrate	22	g
Dietary Fiber	6	g
Sugars	2	g
Protein	8	g

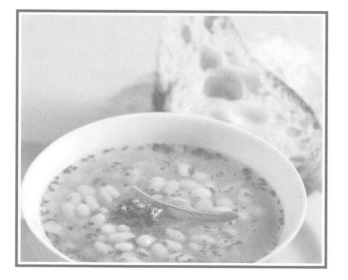

Pasta

Baked Macaroni and Cheese, 83

Beef Stroganoff, 84

Corkscrew Pasta with Sage and Peppers, 85

Eggplant Lasagna, 86

Fettucine Verde with Tomato Sauce, 87

Fettucine with Peppers and Broccoli, 88

Garlic Fettucine, 89

Linguine with Clam Sauce, 90

Linguine with Garlic Broccoli Sauce, 91

Pasta with Vegetable Clam Sauce, 92

Rigatoni with Chicken and Three-Pepper Sauce, 93

Spaghetti Pie, 94

Spaghetti with Pesto Sauce, 95

Stuffed Manicotti, 96

Vegetable Lo Mein, 97

Baked Macaroni and Cheese

This version is creamy and oh, so tasty.

1 cup uncooked elbow macaroni
1/2 cup egg substitute
1 cup evaporated fat-free milk
1 cup small curd low-fat cottage cheese

1/4 cup shredded sharp Cheddar cheese
Dash salt
Fresh ground pepper
1 Tbsp Dijon mustard
1 Tbsp dried bread crumbs

1. Prepare macaroni according to package directions (without adding salt). Drain and set aside.
2. In a large mixing bowl, combine the remaining ingredients except the bread crumbs with the cooked macaroni.
3. Coat a 1-quart baking dish with cooking spray and spoon the mixture into the dish. Sprinkle the top with bread crumbs. Bake at 350 degrees for 1 hour and serve hot.

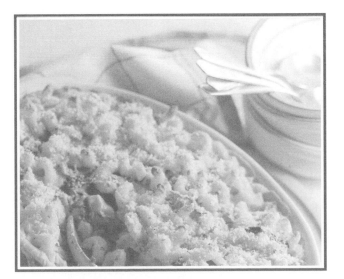

Beef Stroganoff

This casserole is hearty, tasty, and never goes out of style.

1 Tbsp canola oil
2 Tbsp minced onion
1 1/2 lb lean sirloin steak, trimmed
    of fat, thinly sliced, and cut into
    bite-sized pieces

1/2 lb fresh mushrooms, sliced
Fresh ground pepper
Dash nutmeg
1 cup fat-free sour cream
4 cups cooked noodles, hot

1. In a large skillet over medium-high heat, heat the oil. Add the onion, beef, and mushrooms and sauté for 5 minutes or until desired degree of doneness. Add the pepper and nutmeg.
2. Reduce the heat to low and add the sour cream, stirring constantly until well blended.
3. Place noodles on a serving dish and place beef mixture on top. Serve.

NUTRITION FACTS
8 Servings
**Serving Size 2–3 oz meat
  plus 1/2 cup noodles**

AMOUNT PER SERVING

Exchanges
2 Starch
2 Lean Meat

Calories	279
Calories from Fat	58
Total Fat	6 g
Saturated Fat	2 g
Cholesterol	67 mg
Sodium	59 mg
Total Carbohydrate	27 g
Dietary Fiber	1 g
Sugars	3 g
Protein	24 g

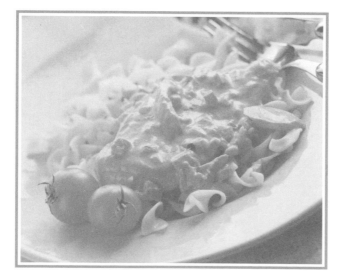

Corkscrew Pasta with Sage and Peppers

This dish is simple to prepare and pretty to serve.

2 Tbsp chicken broth
1 garlic clove, minced
1/2 cup chopped onion
1/2 each red, green, and yellow bell peppers, cut into thin strips
2 Tbsp chopped fresh sage

1 15-oz can tomato puree
1 Tbsp tomato paste
2 Tbsp red wine
1 tsp crushed red pepper (optional)
1 lb cooked corkscrew pasta (or any other shaped pasta)

1. In a large skillet over medium heat, heat broth. Add garlic and onion and sauté for 5 to 8 minutes. Add peppers and sauté for another 7 minutes.

2. Add sage, tomato puree, tomato paste, red wine, and red pepper. Lower heat to a simmer and cook for 15 minutes.

3. Add cooked pasta and let stand for 5 minutes. Serve.

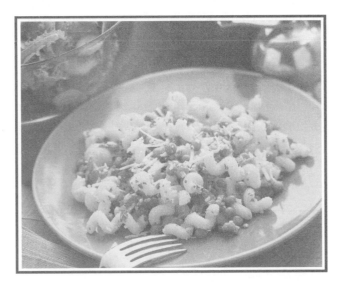

Eggplant Lasagna

Layers of tender eggplant replace noodles in this hearty entree that can be made ahead and frozen.

1 3/4 cups chopped onion
2 medium garlic cloves, minced
1 14.5-oz can diced tomatoes, undrained
5 Tbsp tomato paste
1/2 cup water
2 Tbsp fresh chopped parsley
1 tsp oregano
1/2 tsp dried basil
Fresh ground pepper
1 large eggplant, peeled and sliced into 1/4-inch slices
1 cup shredded fat-free mozzarella cheese
1 cup low-fat cottage cheese
4 Tbsp grated fresh Parmesan cheese

1. Coat a large skillet with nonstick cooking spray. Add onion and garlic and sauté over low heat until onion is tender, about 6 minutes.

2. Stir in tomatoes, tomato paste, water, parsley, oregano, basil, and pepper. Bring mixture to a boil. Reduce heat and simmer, covered, for 30 minutes, stirring occasionally.

3. To steam eggplant slices, place 1 inch of water in a large pot. Arrange eggplant slices on a steamer, cover pot, and steam until eggplant is tender, about 5 minutes. Do not overcook.

4. Combine mozzarella and cottage cheeses together and set aside.

5. Coat a 13 × 9 × 2-inch baking pan with cooking spray and place half of the eggplant in the pan. Top eggplant with half of the cheese mixture and half of the sauce, and sprinkle with half of the Parmesan cheese. Repeat.

6. Bake at 350 degrees for 30 to 35 minutes, and serve hot.

Fettucine Verde with Tomato Sauce

You probably have these ingredients in your cupboard right now.

1/4 lb uncooked spinach fettucine
2/3 cup fat-free ricotta cheese
1/2 cup canned tomatoes
1 large garlic clove, minced

1 small onion, finely chopped
1/4 tsp dried oregano
1/2 tsp dried basil
1 Tbsp Parmesan cheese

1. Prepare the pasta according to package directions (without adding salt), drain, and rinse thoroughly.
2. Place the pasta in a 1-quart casserole dish, and spoon ricotta cheese in center of pasta. Cover and bake at 300 degrees for 8 to 10 minutes until ricotta is heated through.
3. In a small saucepan, combine the tomatoes with the remaining ingredients, bring to a boil, reduce the heat, and let simmer for 3 to 5 minutes or until onion is tender.
4. Remove pasta from oven, and spoon sauce around ricotta cheese. Sprinkle Parmesan cheese over all and serve.

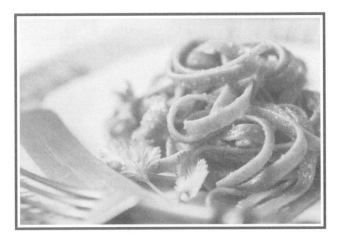

Fettucine with Peppers and Broccoli

This light pasta entree is loaded with Vitamin C-rich vegetables.

2 Tbsp olive oil
2 medium garlic cloves, minced
2 large red bell peppers, halved,
   seeded, and cut into 1/2-inch
   strips

8 oz uncooked fettucine
1 1/2 lb fresh broccoli
1/4 cup Parmesan cheese

1. In a large skillet over medium heat, heat the olive oil. Add the garlic and sauté for 1 minute. Add the peppers and continue sautéing for 3 to 5 minutes or until peppers are just tender, stirring occasionally. Remove from heat and set aside.

2. Prepare the fettucine according to package directions (without adding salt) and drain. Wash the broccoli and peel the tough stalks (if necessary). To a large pot of boiling water, add the broccoli and then turn off the heat. After 1 minute, rinse the broccoli under cold running water to stop the cooking process, then drain. (This method of blanching helps the broccoli to retain its bright green color and crispness.)

3. In a large bowl, toss the fettucine with the peppers, and arrange the broccoli on top. Sprinkle with Parmesan cheese and serve.

NUTRITION FACTS
4 Servings
Serving Size 1 cup

AMOUNT PER SERVING

Exchanges
3 Starch
2 Vegetable
1 1/2 Fat

Calories	362	
Calories from Fat	102	
Total Fat	11	g
Saturated Fat	2	g
Cholesterol*	58	mg
Sodium	142	mg
Total Carbohydrate	51	g
Dietary Fiber	7	g
Sugars	6	g
Protein	15	g

*If the fettucine is made without egg, the cholesterol count is zero.

NUTRITION FACTS

5 Servings
Serving Size 1 cup

AMOUNT PER SERVING

Exchanges
2 Starch
1 Vegetable
1 Fat

Calories	240
Calories from Fat	71
Total Fat	8 g
Saturated Fat	1 g
Cholesterol*	32 mg
Sodium	51 mg
with added salt	147 mg
Total Carbohydrate	38 g
Dietary Fiber	4 g
Sugars	10 g
Protein	7 g

*If the fettucine is made
 without egg, the cholesterol
 count is zero.

Garlic Fettucine

This is a great dish for garlic lovers!

2 Tbsp olive oil
12 plum tomatoes, seeded and diced
4 cloves garlic, minced
1/4 tsp salt (optional)
Fresh ground pepper

1 tsp capers
2 tsp chopped black olives
6 oz uncooked fettucine
1/4 cup chopped fresh basil
Parsley sprigs for garnish

1. In a large saucepan over medium heat, heat the oil. Add the tomatoes, garlic, salt, pepper, capers, and olives. Let simmer over low heat for 30 minutes, stirring occasionally.

2. Prepare the fettucine according to package directions (without adding salt) and drain. Transfer the fettucine to a serving bowl and spoon sauce and chopped basil on top. Garnish with parsley sprigs to serve.

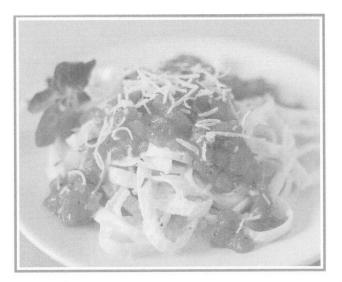

Linguine with Clam Sauce

Try this good red clam sauce recipe with other types of pasta or over rice.

1/2 cup finely chopped onion
1/2 cup finely chopped celery
3 medium garlic cloves, minced
1 7-oz can clams, minced and
  drained, reserve juice
1 15-oz can whole tomatoes,
  undrained and chopped

1/2 tsp dried basil
1/4 tsp dried oregano
1/2 tsp hot pepper sauce
1/3 cup finely minced parsley
2 cups cooked linguine, hot

1. Coat a large saucepan with nonstick cooking spray; place over medium heat until hot. Sauté the onion, celery, and garlic until tender.

2. Add reserved clam juice, tomatoes, basil, oregano, and hot pepper sauce to saucepan. Bring to a boil; reduce heat and let simmer, uncovered, for 35 minutes.

3. Stir in clams and parsley; let simmer for 15 to 20 minutes, or until heated through. Place linguine on a platter, spoon sauce over the pasta, and serve.

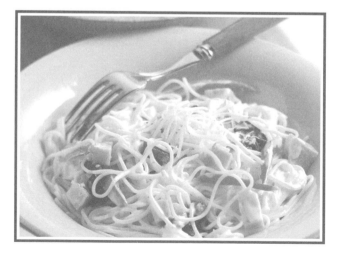

4 Servings
Serving Size 4 oz sauce with
  1/2 cup linguine

AMOUNT PER SERVING

Exchanges
1 1/2 Starch
2 Vegetable

Calories	170
Calories from Fat	12
Total Fat	1 g
Saturated Fat	0 g
Cholesterol	15 mg
Sodium	287 mg
Total Carbohydrate	29 g
Dietary Fiber	3 g
Sugars	7 g
Protein	11 g

Linguine with Garlic Broccoli Sauce

White wine adds a special touch to this pasta dish.

3 Tbsp olive oil
8 medium garlic cloves, minced
Fresh ground pepper
1/4 cup dry white wine
1 tsp dried oregano
1 tsp dried basil

1/2 tsp dried thyme
2 cups broccoli florets
1 lb uncooked linguine or penne
1/4 cup Parmesan cheese
2 Tbsp pine nuts, toasted

1. In a medium skillet over medium heat, heat the oil. Add the garlic and pepper, sautéing for 5 minutes. Add the wine and bring to a boil. Reduce the heat and simmer for 3 to 4 minutes. Add the oregano, basil, and thyme.

2. To a large pot of boiling water, add the broccoli florets and then turn off the heat. After 1 minute, rinse the broccoli under cold running water to stop the cooking process, then drain. (This method of blanching helps the broccoli to retain its bright green color and crispness.) Add the broccoli to the wine sauce and heat 2 more minutes.

3. Prepare the linguine according to package directions (without adding salt) and drain. Transfer the linguine to a large serving bowl and pour the wine sauce over the top. Sprinkle with Parmesan cheese and pine nuts to serve.

Pasta with Vegetable Clam Sauce

This recipe works best with a shaped pasta like rigatoni or shells, so the vegetables stick to the pasta.

5 medium cloves garlic, crushed
2 Tbsp olive oil
4 celery stalks, chopped
2 small zucchini, thinly sliced
4 scallions, chopped
1/4 lb fresh mushrooms, sliced
2 Tbsp chopped fresh parsley

1 7-oz can clams, undrained
2 small tomatoes, chopped
1/3 cup dry white wine
2 Tbsp fresh lemon juice
Fresh ground pepper
1 lb cooked, shaped pasta
Parmesan cheese (optional)

1. In a large skillet over medium heat, heat the oil. Sauté the garlic until lightly browned. Add celery, zucchini, scallions, mushrooms, and parsley; sauté until vegetables are just tender (about 5 minutes).

2. Add clams with their juice, tomatoes, wine, lemon juice, and pepper; stir well. Let simmer, uncovered, for 4 to 5 minutes. Place cooked pasta on a serving platter. Remove sauce from heat and spoon over the pasta. Sprinkle with cheese and serve.

NUTRITION FACTS

8 Servings
Serving Size 1/2 cup pasta plus sauce

AMOUNT PER SERVING

Exchanges
1 Starch
1 Vegetable
1 Fat

Calories	162	
Total Fat	5	g
Saturated Fat	1	g
Calories from Fat	42	
Cholesterol	10	mg
Total Carbohydrate	22	g
Dietary Fiber	2	g
Sugars	5	g
Protein	8	g
Sodium	94	mg

NUTRITION FACTS

8 Servings
Serving Size 1/2 chicken
breast and 1 cup pasta
with pepper sauce

AMOUNT PER SERVING

Exchanges
3 Starch
1 Vegetable
3 Lean Meat

Calories	448
Calories from Fat	100
Total Fat	11 g
Saturated Fat	2 g
Cholesterol	72 mg
Sodium	78 mg
with added salt	94 mg
Total Carbohydrate	50 g
Dietary Fiber	3 g
Sugars	6 g
Protein	35 g

Rigatoni with Chicken and Three-Pepper Sauce

This dish is slightly spicy and very colorful!

16 oz uncooked rigatoni (or substitute any other shaped pasta)
1/4 cup olive oil
1 medium onion, chopped
1 large green bell pepper, julienned
1 large red bell pepper, julienned
1 large yellow bell pepper, julienned
2 garlic cloves, minced
2 tomatoes, chopped

1/2 cup low-sodium chicken broth
1/4 cup minced parsley
1/2 tsp dried basil
Dash salt and pepper (optional)
Dash crushed red pepper
2 Tbsp lemon juice
4 boneless, skinless chicken breasts, halved and cooked

1. Cook the rigatoni according to package directions (without adding salt), drain, and set aside. In a large skillet over medium heat, heat the oil. Add the onion, peppers, and garlic and sauté for 6 minutes.

2. Add the tomatoes, chicken broth, parsley, basil, salt, pepper, and crushed red pepper. Add lemon juice. Add chicken to the skillet and cook chicken in sauce over low heat just until chicken is warmed in the sauce.

3. Arrange the cooked rigatoni on a serving platter. Spoon chicken and pepper sauce over rigatoni and serve.

Spaghetti Pie

This is a great way to use leftover spaghetti.

4 cups cooked spaghetti
  (about 1/2 lb dry)
2 egg whites
2 Tbsp fat-free milk
1/4 cup grated fresh Parmesan
  cheese

1 tsp dried oregano
1 tsp dried basil
1 tsp paprika
1/2 tsp rosemary

1. In a medium bowl, combine all ingredients and mix well.
2. Pour spaghetti mixture into an ovenproof nonstick round casserole dish or skillet and spread evenly.
3. Bake pie, uncovered, at 350 degrees until golden brown, about 20 minutes. Cut into wedges and serve.

NUTRITION FACTS

4 Servings
Serving Size about 1 cup

AMOUNT PER SERVING

Exchanges
3 Starch

Calories	232	
Calories from Fat	23	
Total Fat	3	g
Saturated Fat	1	g
Cholesterol	4	mg
Sodium	126	mg
Total Carbohydrate	40	g
Dietary Fiber	2	g
Sugars	2	g
Protein	11	g

Spaghetti with Pesto Sauce

Fresh basil, garlic, cheese, and pine nuts turn everyday spaghetti into something special.

3 cups fresh basil, stems removed
3 garlic cloves, chopped
1/4 cup olive oil
3/4 cup pine nuts, toasted

1/4 cup Parmesan cheese
Fresh ground pepper
1 lb cooked spaghetti, hot

1. Wash and dry basil. Place basil in a blender or food processor with garlic, olive oil, pine nuts, cheese, and pepper and process until smooth.
2. Transfer cooked spaghetti to a serving bowl. Add pesto and toss thoroughly to serve.

Stuffed Manicotti

You can also use this filling for lasagna or stuffed shells.

2 Tbsp low-sodium chicken broth
1/2 cup minced onion
1/2 cup minced carrot
1 garlic clove, minced
1 cup low-fat ricotta cheese
1/4 cup egg substitute

2 Tbsp Parmesan cheese
1 Tbsp chopped fresh basil
8 large manicotti shells, cooked
2 cups Marinara Sauce (see recipe, page 31)

1. In a skillet over medium heat, heat broth. Add onion, carrot, and garlic and sauté for 5 to 7 minutes, until onion is tender.
2. In a large bowl, combine vegetables with ricotta cheese, egg substitute, Parmesan cheese, and basil. Mix well.
3. Stuff some of the mixture into each shell. Place stuffed manicotti shells in a large casserole dish. Pour marinara sauce on top, and let cook at 350 degrees for 20 minutes.

NUTRITION FACTS

4 Servings
Serving Size 2 stuffed manicotti

AMOUNT PER SERVING

Exchanges
2 1/2 Starch
1 Vegetable
1 Lean Meat

Calories	275	
Calories from Fat	34	
Total Fat	4	g
Saturated Fat	2	g
Cholesterol	27	mg
Sodium	458	mg
Total Carbohydrate	45	g
Dietary Fiber	3	g
Sugars	8	g
Protein	18	g

Vegetable Lo Mein

Restaurant-style lo mein has far too much fat to be considered healthy, so make this lower-fat version instead.

1 cup plus 2 Tbsp low-sodium chicken broth
2 garlic cloves, minced
1/4 cup minced scallions
2 tsp grated fresh ginger
2 carrots, peeled and cut into 1/4-inch slices
3 celery stalks, cut on the diagonal into 1/4-inch slices
1/2 cup sliced mushrooms
1 1/2 cups broccoli florets
2 Tbsp dry sherry
1 Tbsp lite soy sauce
1 tsp sesame oil
1 Tbsp cornstarch
1/2 lb cooked vermicelli

1. In a large skillet or wok, heat 2 Tbsp of broth. Add garlic, scallions, and ginger and sauté for 30 seconds.

2. Add carrots, celery, and mushrooms and sauté for 5 minutes. Add broccoli and 1/2 cup of broth, cover, and steam for 5 minutes.

3. In a small bowl, combine the remaining 1/2 cup of broth with sherry, soy sauce, and sesame oil. Add cornstarch and mix well.

4. Remove cover and add cornstarch mixture. Cook for 1 minute more until mixture thickens. Toss in cooked noodles and mix well. Serve.

Poultry

Apple-Glazed Cornish Hens, 101

Baked Chicken and Peas, 102

Baked Chicken Breasts Supreme, 103

Baked Chicken Kiev, 104

Baked Chicken with Wine Sauce, 105

Baked Lemon Chicken, 106

Chicken and Shrimp, 107

Chicken and Zucchini, 108

Chicken Dijon, 109

Chicken Paprika, 110

Chicken Parmesan, 111

Chicken Provençal, 112

Chicken Rose Marie, 113

Chicken with Cream Sauce, 114

Chicken with Green Peppercorn Sauce, 115

Grilled Chicken with Garlic, 116

Grilled Lemon Mustard Chicken, 117

Herbed Cornish Hens, 118

Indoor Barbecued Turkey, 119

Marinated Chicken Kabobs, 120

Mushroom Chicken, 121

Oven-Baked Chicken Tenders, 122

Poached Chicken with Bay Leaves, 123

Sautéed Chicken with Artichoke Hearts, 124

Spicy Chicken Drumsticks, 125

Summer Chicken Kabobs, 126

Turkey Burgers, 127

Turkey Cutlets Diane, 128

Turkey with Almond Duxelles, 129

Apple-Glazed Cornish Hens

This is a great dish to prepare during the holiday season as an alternative to turkey.

4 Cornish hens
12 oz unsweetened apple juice
  concentrate, undiluted
3 Tbsp water

1 Tbsp cornstarch
1 tsp cinnamon
1 medium lemon, sliced

1. Remove giblets from hens and discard. Rinse hens under cold water and pat dry. Using a long, sharp knife, split the hens lengthwise. You may also buy precut hens.

2. Place the hens, cavity side up, in a roasting pan. Dilute 1/2 cup of the apple juice concentrate with the water. Pour juice over the hens. Bake uncovered at 350 degrees for 45 minutes. Turn breast side up.

3. In a small pan over medium heat, combine the remaining apple juice concentrate, cornstarch, and cinnamon; mix well. Add 4 lemon slices and continue cooking until thickened.

4. Remove from heat and brush hens with the sauce. Return the hens to the oven and continue to bake for an additional 15 minutes. Transfer the hens to a serving platter and garnish with remaining lemon slices.

Baked Chicken and Peas

Just add a salad, and you have dinner.

1 Tbsp olive oil
2 Tbsp lite soy sauce
1 1/2 tsp paprika
1/2 tsp dried basil
1/2 tsp dried thyme

4 chicken thighs, skinned
1/4 lb fresh mushrooms, sliced
1/2 cup low-sodium chicken broth
10 oz frozen peas, thawed and
   drained

1. In a shallow 2-quart casserole dish, combine oil, soy sauce, paprika, basil, and thyme. Add chicken thighs, and coat the chicken well.

2. Add mushrooms and chicken broth.

3. Cover and bake at 350 degrees for 50 minutes. Add peas; cover and continue baking for an additional 10 to 15 minutes or until peas are just tender. Remove from oven and serve hot.

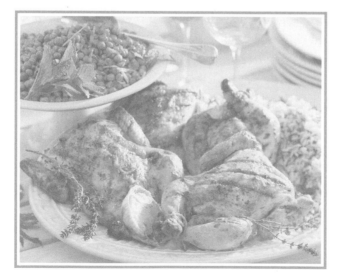

Baked Chicken Breasts Supreme

This is an especially nice dish that is slightly rich without the worry of excess fat. You'll need to start it the night before.

6 3-oz boneless, skinless chicken breast halves
2 cups fat-free sour cream
1/4 cup lemon juice
4 tsp Worcestershire sauce
1 tsp celery salt
2 tsp paprika

1 garlic clove, minced
Dash salt
Fresh ground pepper
1 3/4 cups dried bread crumbs
2 Tbsp olive oil
Parsley sprigs
1 lemon, sliced

1. Wash chicken breasts under cold running water and pat dry. Combine sour cream, lemon juice, Worcestershire sauce, celery salt, paprika, garlic, salt, and pepper. Measure out 1/2 cup of marinade and reserve the rest in the refrigerator.

2. Add chicken to the 1/2 cup of marinade and coat each piece well. Refrigerate overnight. Remove chicken from the marinade, discard marinade, and roll chicken in bread crumbs, coating evenly.

3. Arrange in a single layer in a large baking pan. Drizzle olive oil over the chicken breasts. Bake the chicken at 350 degrees, uncovered, for 45 minutes, or until chicken is no longer pink.

4. Transfer to a serving platter, and serve with remaining marinade as a sauce and parsley and lemon slices as garnish.

Baked Chicken Kiev

This low-fat version of a classic dish is great to serve when entertaining.

6 Tbsp reduced-fat margarine
3 Tbsp minced fresh parsley
1/2 tsp dried rosemary
1/4 tsp garlic powder
Fresh ground pepper

3 whole boneless, skinless chicken
  breasts, halved
1/4 cup fat-free milk
1/3 cup dried bread crumbs
1 lemon, cut into wedges

1. Combine margarine, parsley, rosemary, garlic powder, and pepper in a small mixing bowl. Shape margarine mixture into six 2-inch-long sticks; freeze until firm.

2. Place each chicken breast half between 2 sheets of waxed paper and flatten to 1/4-inch thickness with a meat mallet or rolling pin.

3. Place 1 margarine stick in the center of each chicken breast; fold ends over margarine and roll up, beginning with long side. Secure each end with wooden toothpicks.

4. Dip chicken rolls into the milk and coat thoroughly with bread crumbs. Bake at 400 degrees for 25 minutes until browned.

5. Arrange chicken on a serving platter, spoon juices from pan over the top, garnish with lemon wedges, and serve.

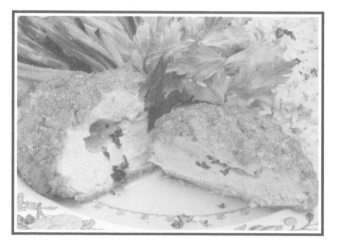

NUTRITION FACTS
6 Servings
Serving Size 3–4 oz

AMOUNT PER SERVING

Exchanges
4 Lean Meat

Calories	219
Calories from Fat	81
Total Fat	9 g
Saturated Fat	2 g
Cholesterol	73 mg
Sodium	210 mg
Total Carbohydrate	5 g
Dietary Fiber	0 g
Sugars	1 g
Protein	28 g

Baked Chicken with Wine Sauce

This wine sauce is also delicious with turkey or Cornish game hens.

4 Tbsp reduced-fat margarine (divided use)

4 whole boneless, skinless chicken breasts, halved

3 Tbsp flour

1/2 cup low-sodium chicken broth

3/4 cup low-fat sour cream

1/4 cup dry white wine

2 tsp grated lemon rind

1 tsp salt (optional)

Fresh ground pepper

1 tsp minced fresh thyme

1/2 tsp ground sage

1/2 cup sliced mushrooms

Fresh parsley sprigs

1. Preheat the oven to 350 degrees. Melt 2 Tbsp of the margarine in a shallow baking dish; place chicken breasts in the dish. Bake uncovered for 30 minutes.

2. Meanwhile, melt remaining margarine in a saucepan, add the flour, and stir until smooth. Add the chicken broth and stir until mixture is thickened. Add the sour cream, wine, lemon rind, salt, pepper, thyme, and sage. Stir until completely smooth.

3. Remove the chicken from the oven and turn the chicken breasts over. Cover the chicken with the mushrooms and pour the sauce over the top. Continue to bake, uncovered, for another 30 minutes or until chicken is no longer pink. Transfer chicken to serving platter, spoon sauce over the chicken, garnish with parsley sprigs, and serve.

Baked Lemon Chicken

This very light chicken dish is great on a spring or summer night.

3 Tbsp lemon juice
1 tsp fresh lemon zest
1 Tbsp finely chopped onion
1/4 tsp paprika
2 Tbsp olive oil

Dash salt
Fresh ground pepper
2 whole boneless, skinless chicken
  breasts, halved

1. Preheat the oven to 400 degrees. In a small bowl, combine all ingredients except chicken.

2. Place chicken in a shallow baking dish and pour lemon mixture over it. Bake for 45 minutes until chicken is no longer pink.

3. Transfer chicken to a serving platter, spoon juices over it, and serve.

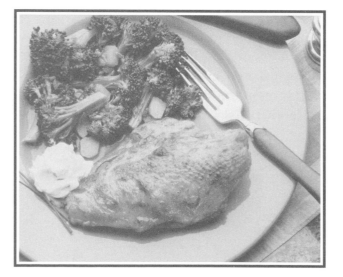

NUTRITION FACTS
4 Servings
Serving Size 3 oz

AMOUNT PER SERVING

Exchanges
3 Lean Meat
1/2 Fat

Calories	205	
Calories from Fat	88	
Total Fat	10	g
Saturated Fat	2	g
Cholesterol	72	mg
Sodium	100	mg
Total Carbohydrate	1	g
Dietary Fiber	0	g
Sugars	0	g
Protein	27	g

Chicken and Shrimp

This skillet dinner cooks nicely while you prepare
a salad and crusty bread.

1 Tbsp olive oil
2 medium onions, chopped
2 garlic cloves, minced
1 cup chopped celery
1 green bell pepper, chopped
2/3 cup uncooked rice

2 cups low-sodium chicken broth
1 1/2 cups cubed precooked chicken
1 16-oz can stewed tomatoes
4 oz shrimp, shelled and deveined
1 tsp hot pepper sauce
Fresh ground pepper

1. Coat a large skillet with the oil and heat over medium heat. Add onion, garlic, celery, and green pepper; sauté until tender.

2. Stir in the rice, broth, chicken, and tomatoes. Bring to a boil, reduce the heat, and let simmer for 25 minutes.

3. Add the shrimp, hot pepper sauce, and pepper and let simmer for 5 minutes. Transfer to a serving platter to serve.

Chicken and Zucchini

Here's a quick stir-fry dish with a hint of ginger.

1 Tbsp olive oil
4 whole boneless, skinless chicken breasts, cut into thin strips about 1/8 inch wide
2 garlic cloves, minced
1 tsp grated fresh ginger

1 Tbsp lite soy sauce
1/3 cup sliced celery
1/2 cup sliced fresh mushrooms
1 cup julienned zucchini
2 tsp cornstarch
3 Tbsp water

1. Heat the oil in a large skillet or wok. Add the chicken, garlic, and ginger. Stir-fry until chicken turns white, about 5 minutes.

2. Stir in the soy sauce, celery, mushrooms, and zucchini. Cover and continue to cook for about 5 minutes.

3. Add the cornstarch to the water and slowly add this mixture to the chicken, stirring constantly. Continue to cook for 2 to 5 minutes until mixture is thickened. Remove from heat and serve.

NUTRITION FACTS
8 Servings
Serving Size 3–4 oz

AMOUNT PER SERVING

Exchanges
3 Lean Meat

Calories	165
Calories from Fat	43
Total Fat	5 g
Saturated Fat	1 g
Cholesterol	72 mg
Sodium	143 mg
Total Carbohydrate	2 g
Dietary Fiber	0 g
Sugars	1 g
Protein	27 g

Chicken Dijon

Add colorful vegetables and wild rice for a complete meal.

4 whole boneless, skinless chicken breasts, halved
1 Tbsp olive oil
1/4 cup minced onion
2 cups sliced fresh mushrooms
2 garlic cloves, minced

1/4 cup dry white wine
1/2 cup low-sodium chicken broth
4 Tbsp minced fresh parsley
Fresh ground pepper
1 Tbsp Dijon mustard

1. Place chicken breasts between 2 sheets of waxed paper; flatten to 1/4 inch using a meat mallet. Coat a large skillet with nonstick cooking spray and place over medium-high heat; heat until hot.

2. Add chicken to the skillet and cook for 2 to 3 minutes until chicken is browned on each side. Remove chicken from skillet; set aside and keep warm.

3. In the same pan, add the olive oil. Sauté the onion, mushrooms, and garlic for 2 to 3 minutes. Add the wine, chicken broth, and 2 Tbsp of the parsley and cook for 3 to 4 minutes.

4. Add the chicken back to the pan and cook over medium heat for 10 to 12 minutes. Remove chicken and vegetables using a slotted spoon. Arrange the chicken on a serving platter and keep warm.

5. Continue cooking broth mixture until it is reduced to 1/3 cup. Remove from heat and whisk in the remaining parsley, pepper, and mustard. Spoon sauce over the chicken and serve.

Chicken Paprika

This version of a classic Hungarian dish is much lower in fat.

1 Tbsp olive oil
1 large onion, minced
1 medium red bell pepper, julienned
1 cup sliced fresh mushrooms
1 cup water
1–2 tsp paprika

2 Tbsp lemon juice
Dash salt
Fresh ground pepper
4 whole boneless, skinless chicken
  breasts, halved
8 oz low-fat sour cream

1. Heat oil in a large skillet. Add onion, red pepper, and mushrooms and sauté until tender, about 3 to 4 minutes.
2. Add water, paprika, lemon juice, salt, and pepper, blending well. Add chicken; cover and let simmer for 25 to 30 minutes or until chicken is no longer pink.
3. Stir in the sour cream and continue to cook for 1 to 2 minutes. Do not boil. Serve hot.

NUTRITION FACTS

8 Servings
Serving Size 3 oz

AMOUNT PER SERVING

Exchanges
1/2 Starch
1 Vegetable
3 Lean Meat

Calories	218
Calories from Fat	62
Total Fat	7 g
Saturated Fat	2 g
Cholesterol	72 mg
Sodium	123 mg
Total Carbohydrate	9 g
Dietary Fiber	1 g
Sugars	6 g
Protein	29 g

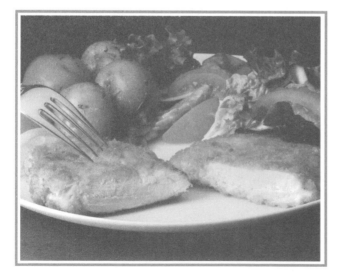

NUTRITION FACTS

6 Servings
Serving Size 3 oz

AMOUNT PER SERVING

Exchanges
3 Very Lean Meat
1 1/2 Fat

Calories	181
Calories from Fat	56
Total Fat	6 g
Saturated Fat	1 g
Cholesterol	51 mg
Sodium	151 mg
Total Carbohydrate	4 g
Dietary Fiber	1 g
Sugars	1 g
Protein	21 g

Chicken Parmesan

Here's an all-time favorite that creates an enticing aroma.

6 3-oz boneless, skinless chicken breasts halves

1/2 cup Homemade Seasoned Bread Crumbs (see recipe, page 223)

2 Tbsp grated fresh Parmesan cheese

1 tsp dried oregano

Fresh ground pepper (optional)

1/2 cup egg substitute

1 1/2 Tbsp olive oil

1 cup dry white wine

1. Pound the chicken breasts until thin.

2. Combine the bread crumbs, Parmesan cheese, oregano, and pepper; set aside.

3. Beat the egg substitute in a shallow dish. Dip the chicken breasts into the egg and then the crumb mixture, coating both sides.

4. Heat the oil in a large nonstick skillet, add chicken, and sauté until golden brown, about 4 to 5 minutes on each side or until chicken is no longer pink. Remove chicken and set aside on a platter.

5. Drain fat from the skillet and add the wine, bringing the mixture to a boil while scraping down residue from the skillet. Pour sauce over the chicken and serve.

Chicken Provençal

Your guests will love this fast, easy-to-prepare dish.

2 Tbsp olive oil

1 tsp dried basil

2 whole boneless, skinless chicken breasts, halved

1 medium garlic clove, minced

1/4 cup minced onion

1/4 cup minced green bell pepper

1/2 cup dry white wine

1 8-oz can chopped tomatoes

1/4 cup pitted black olives

Fresh ground pepper

1. Heat the oil in a skillet over medium heat. Stir in basil, add chicken, and brown about 3 to 5 minutes.

2. Add the remaining ingredients and cook uncovered over medium heat for 20 minutes or until chicken is no longer pink. Transfer to serving platter and season with additional pepper before serving.

NUTRITION FACTS

4 Servings
Serving Size 3–4 oz

AMOUNT PER SERVING

Exchanges
1 Vegetable
4 Lean Meat

Calories	240	
Calories from Fat	98	
Total Fat	11	g
Saturated Fat	2	g
Cholesterol	72	mg
Sodium	294	mg
Total Carbohydrate	5	g
Dietary Fiber	1	g
Sugars	4	g
Protein	27	g

Chicken Rose Marie

Try serving this dish with orzo (a rice-shaped pasta) and good, crusty French bread.

3 whole boneless, skinless chicken breasts, halved
1 cup dried bread crumbs
1/4 cup olive oil
1/4 cup low-sodium chicken broth
Grated zest of 1 lemon
3 medium garlic cloves, minced
1/4 cup minced fresh parsley
1/2 cup fresh lemon juice
1/2 cup water
1/2 tsp dried oregano
1 medium lemon, cut into wedges
Parsley sprigs

1. Rinse the chicken in cold water and then roll it in bread crumbs. Spray a skillet with nonstick cooking spray and brown the coated chicken breasts over medium heat about 3 minutes on each side. Transfer the browned chicken to a baking dish.

2. In a small bowl, combine the remaining ingredients, except the lemon and parsley. Pour the sauce over the chicken. Bake the chicken at 325 degrees, uncovered, for 30 minutes until chicken is no longer pink.

3. Transfer to a serving platter and spoon sauce over the chicken. Garnish with lemon and parsley.

Chicken with Cream Sauce

This dish is good with steamed green beans or asparagus.

1 Tbsp canola oil

4 3-oz boneless, skinless chicken breast halves

1/2 cup sliced mushrooms

3 Tbsp flour

1/2 cup low-sodium chicken broth

3/4 cup white wine

2 tsp lemon zest

1/2 tsp lemon pepper

1 cup fat-free sour cream

Parsley sprigs

1. In a large nonstick skillet, heat the oil; add chicken and cook for 5 minutes on each side. Remove chicken and keep warm. Add mushrooms to skillet and cook until tender.

2. In a small bowl, whisk flour with broth and wine. Stir mixture into skillet and add lemon zest and pepper. Cook until thickened and bubbly.

3. Return chicken to skillet and cook until chicken is no longer pink. Transfer chicken to a platter. Stir sour cream into skillet and heat thoroughly. Pour sauce over chicken and garnish with parsley.

NUTRITION FACTS

4 Servings
Serving Size 3 oz

AMOUNT PER SERVING

Exchanges
1/2 Carbohydrate
4 Very Lean Meat
1 Fat

Calories	260
Calories from Fat	62
Total Fat	7 g
Saturated Fat	1 g
Cholesterol	79 mg
Sodium	156 mg
Total Carbohydrate	8 g
Dietary Fiber	0 g
Sugars	3 g
Protein	32 g

Chicken with Green Peppercorn Sauce

This is a quick dish to fix when unexpected guests drop by.

1 Tbsp olive oil
4 3-oz boneless, skinless chicken
   breast halves
2 scallions, sliced
1 Tbsp flour
1/2 cup fat-free half-and-half

1/4 cup low-sodium chicken broth
1/4 cup dry white wine
1 tsp green peppercorns, drained
   (or 1 tsp dried green peppercorns,
   reconstituted)
1/2 tsp salt (optional)

1. In a large skillet, heat the olive oil over medium heat. Sauté chicken for 5 minutes per side; remove to a platter and keep warm.

2. Sauté scallions for 1 minute and add the flour. Add the half-and-half, chicken broth, wine, peppercorns, and salt. Continue cooking until sauce thickens.

3. Return the chicken to the pan and continue cooking until chicken is no longer pink. Transfer chicken to a platter and serve with sauce.

Grilled Chicken with Garlic

Roasted garlic is the secret to this flavorful chicken dish.

4 3-oz boneless, skinless chicken breast halves

2 Tbsp canola oil (divided use)

1 cup red wine

3 sprigs thyme

5 garlic cloves, minced

5 garlic cloves, whole and unpeeled

Fresh ground pepper

1. In a plastic zippered bag, place chicken, 1 Tbsp oil, wine, thyme, and minced garlic. Marinate for 2 to 3 hours in the refrigerator.

2. Preheat the oven to 375 degrees.

3. Spread whole garlic cloves on a cookie sheet, drizzle with remaining oil, and sprinkle with pepper. Bake for 30 minutes, stirring occasionally, until soft.

4. When cool, squeeze garlic paste from cloves and mash in a small bowl with a fork.

5. Remove chicken from marinade and grill for 12 to 15 minutes, turning frequently and brushing with garlic paste. Transfer to a platter and serve hot.

NUTRITION FACTS

4 Servings
Serving Size 3 oz

AMOUNT PER SERVING

Exchanges
4 Lean Meat

Calories	217	
Calories from Fat	91	
Total Fat	10	g
Saturated Fat	1	g
Cholesterol	73	mg
Sodium	65	mg
Total Carbohydrate	2	g
Dietary Fiber	0	g
Sugars	0	g
Protein	27	g

Grilled Lemon Mustard Chicken

Note that you need to let the chicken marinate overnight in this recipe.

Juice of 6 medium lemons
1/2 cup mustard seeds
1 Tbsp minced fresh tarragon
2 Tbsp fresh ground pepper

4 garlic cloves, minced
2 Tbsp olive oil
3 whole boneless, skinless chicken
   breasts, halved

1. In a small mixing bowl, combine the lemon juice, mustard seeds, tarragon, pepper, garlic, and oil; mix well.
2. Place chicken in a baking dish and pour marinade on top. Cover and refrigerate overnight.
3. Grill chicken over medium heat for 10 to 15 minutes, basting with marinade. Serve hot.

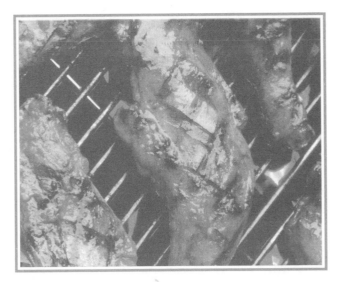

Herbed Cornish Hens

*A perfect blend of herbs and wine complement the
natural flavor of Cornish game hens.*

4 Cornish hens
2 cups light rosé wine
2 garlic cloves, minced
1/2 tsp onion powder
1/2 tsp celery seeds

1/2 tsp poultry seasoning
1/2 tsp paprika
1/2 tsp dried basil
Fresh ground pepper

1. Remove the giblets from the hens; rinse under cold water and pat dry.
   Using a long, sharp knife, split each hen lengthwise. You may also buy
   precut hens.

2. Place the hens, cavity side up, on a rack in a shallow roasting pan. Pour
   1 1/2 cups of the wine over the hens; set aside.

3. In a shallow bowl, combine the garlic, onion powder, celery seeds, poultry seasoning, paprika, basil, and pepper. Sprinkle half the combined
   seasonings over the cavity of each split half. Cover and refrigerate. Allow
   the hens to marinate for 2 to 3 hours.

4. Preheat the oven to 350 degrees. Bake the hens uncovered for 1 hour.
   Remove from oven, turn breast side up, pour remaining 1/2 cup wine
   over the top, and sprinkle with remaining seasonings.

5. Continue to bake for an additional 25 to 30 minutes, basting every 10
   minutes until hens are done. Transfer to a serving platter and serve hot.

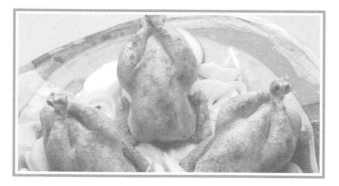

NUTRITION FACTS

8 Servings
Serving Size 4 oz

AMOUNT PER SERVING

Exchanges
4 Lean Meat

Calories	225
Calories from Fat	78
Total Fat	9 g
Saturated Fat	2 g
Cholesterol	103 mg
Sodium	103 mg
Total Carbohydrate	0 g
Dietary Fiber	0 g
Sugars	0 g
Protein	34 g

Indoor Barbecued Turkey

~

Have turkey anytime! Enjoy slowly roasted turkey breast in a beer-mustard sauce.

1 5-lb (including bone) turkey breast
1 Tbsp prepared mustard
1/2 cup lite beer
1/4 cup red wine vinegar
3/4 cup ketchup
1 Tbsp no-added-salt tomato paste
1/2 cup spicy no-added-salt tomato juice (or spice up mild juice with several drops of hot pepper sauce)
Fresh ground pepper

1. Preheat the oven to 350 degrees. Spread turkey breast with mustard. Combine beer, vinegar, ketchup, tomato paste, and tomato juice in a small bowl.

2. Pour mixture over turkey, then sprinkle with pepper. Roast, covered, for 1 1/2 hours. Remove cover and roast an additional 1 hour, basting occasionally. Transfer to a serving platter and serve.

Marinated Chicken Kabobs

These kabobs are great to grill on a hot summer night.

4 tsp fresh lemon juice

1/2 tsp cayenne pepper

Fresh ground pepper

1-inch piece of fresh ginger, peeled and minced

1 tsp curry powder

4 tsp olive oil

2 whole boneless, skinless chicken breasts, halved, cut into 1/4-inch strips

1. In a medium bowl, combine all ingredients except the chicken. Add the chicken and let marinate overnight in the refrigerator.

2. Thread the chicken onto metal or wooden skewers (remember to soak the wooden skewers in water before using).

3. Grill over medium heat until chicken is no longer pink, about 15 minutes. Transfer to a platter and serve.

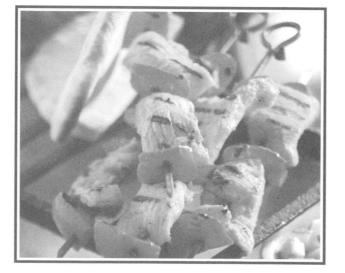

Exchanges
3 Lean Meat

Calories	181
Calories from Fat	66
Total Fat	7 g
Saturated Fat	1 g
Cholesterol	72 mg
Sodium	64 mg
Total Carbohydrate	0 g
Dietary Fiber	0 g
Sugars	0 g
Protein	26 g

Mushroom Chicken

This great dish for leftover chicken is ready in less than 20 minutes.

2 Tbsp canola oil
1/2 cup sliced fresh mushrooms
2 Tbsp flour
Dash salt
Fresh ground pepper
1/3 cup sherry

1 cup fat-free evaporated milk
2 1/2 cups cubed precooked chicken
   breast
1/4 cup white raisins
2 cups precooked rice, hot
1/2 cup toasted slivered almonds

1. In a large skillet, heat oil over medium heat. Add mushrooms and sauté for 3 minutes.
2. Stir in flour, salt, and pepper. Add sherry and cook until sherry has been absorbed.
3. Add milk; cook and stir until thickened and bubbly. Stir in chicken and raisins; let simmer until heated thoroughly.
4. Arrange the rice on a serving platter, spoon chicken mixture over rice, top with slivered almonds, and serve.

Oven-Baked Chicken Tenders

Kids will love these easy-to-eat strips of crunchy chicken that are baked, not fried. Serve with Marinara Sauce (see recipe, page 31).

2 whole boneless, skinless chicken breasts, halved

2 egg whites, beaten

1/2 cup whole-wheat cracker crumbs

1 tsp dried basil

1/2 tsp dried oregano

1/2 tsp dried thyme

1 tsp paprika

2 tsp grated fresh Parmesan cheese

1. Cut each chicken breast into 2 1/2-inch strips.
2. Dip each strip into egg whites.
3. On a flat plate or in a plastic bag, combine cracker crumbs with spices and cheese. Add chicken strips and coat with the crumb mixture.
4. On a nonstick cookie sheet, place chicken strips side by side in one layer. Bake at 350 degrees for 10 to 12 minutes until golden and crunchy.

NUTRITION FACTS

4 Servings
Serving Size 3 oz

AMOUNT PER SERVING

Exchanges
1/2 Starch
3 Lean Meat

Calories	197	
Calories from Fat	46	
Total Fat	5	g
Saturated Fat	1	g
Cholesterol	73	mg
Sodium	181	mg
Total Carbohydrate	6	g
Dietary Fiber	0	g
Sugars	0	g
Protein	29	g

Poached Chicken with Bay Leaves

You'll love this poached chicken, surrounded by tender vegetables in a bay leaf–scented broth.

4 quarts low-sodium chicken broth
2 cups dry white wine
4 large bay leaves
4 sprigs fresh thyme
Dash salt and pepper
1 4-lb chicken, giblets removed, washed and patted dry

1/2 lb carrots, peeled and julienned
1/2 lb turnips, peeled and julienned
1/2 lb parsnips, peeled and julienned
4 small leeks, washed and trimmed

1. In a large stockpot, combine broth, wine, bay leaves, thyme, salt, and pepper. Let simmer over medium heat while you prepare the chicken.
2. Stuff the cavity with 1/3 each of the carrots, turnips, and parsnips; then truss. Add the stuffed chicken to the stockpot and poach, covered, over low heat for 30 minutes.
3. Add remaining vegetables with the leeks and continue to simmer for 25 to 30 minutes, or until juices run clear when the chicken is pierced with a fork.
4. Remove chicken and vegetables to a serving platter. Carve the chicken, remove the skin, and surround the sliced meat with poached vegetables to serve.

Sautéed Chicken with Artichoke Hearts

Fresh tarragon is best with this chicken and artichoke flavor combination.

3 whole boneless, skinless chicken breasts, halved

1/2 cup low-sodium chicken broth

1/4 cup dry white wine

2 8-oz cans artichokes, packed in water, drained and quartered

1 medium onion, diced

1 medium green bell pepper, chopped

1 tsp minced fresh tarragon (or 1/2 tsp dried)

1/4 tsp white pepper

2 tsp cornstarch

1 Tbsp cold water

2 medium tomatoes, cut into wedges

1. Coat a large skillet with nonstick cooking spray; place over medium heat until hot. Add the chicken and sauté until lightly browned, about 3 to 4 minutes per side.

2. Add the chicken broth, wine, artichokes, onion, green pepper, tarragon, and white pepper; stir well. Bring to a boil, cover, reduce heat, and let simmer for 10 to 15 minutes or until chicken is no longer pink and vegetables are just tender.

3. Combine the cornstarch and water; add to chicken mixture along with the tomato wedges, stirring until mixture has thickened. Remove from the heat and serve.

NUTRITION FACTS

6 Servings
Serving Size 3–4 oz chicken with topping

AMOUNT PER SERVING

Exchanges
1 Vegetable
3 Lean Meat

Calories	186	
Calories from Fat	8	
Total Fat	4	g
Saturated Fat	1	g
Cholesterol	73	mg
Sodium	250	mg
Total Carbohydrate	9	g
Dietary Fiber	2	g
Sugars	3	g
Protein	29	g

Spicy Chicken Drumsticks

Serve these as an appetizer on a hot summer day.

1/4 cup plain low-fat yogurt

2 Tbsp hot pepper sauce

4 chicken drumsticks, skinned

1/4 cup dried bread crumbs

1. In a shallow dish, combine yogurt and hot pepper sauce, mixing well. Add drumsticks, turning to coat, cover, and marinate in the refrigerator for 2 to 4 hours.

2. Remove drumsticks from marinade, dredge in bread crumbs, and place in a baking dish. Bake at 350 degrees for 40 to 50 minutes. Transfer to a serving platter and serve.

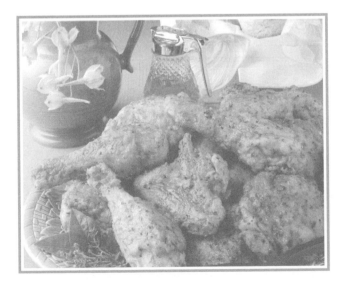

Summer Chicken Kabobs

You can also grill these kabobs in the fall, when squash is in season.

1/4 cup lime juice

2 Tbsp olive oil

1 Tbsp minced parsley

1/2 tsp dried thyme

1 garlic clove, minced

Fresh ground pepper

2 whole boneless, skinless chicken breasts, cubed

1 small yellow squash, cut into 2-inch pieces

1 small zucchini, cut into 1-inch pieces

4 large cherry tomatoes

1. In a shallow dish, combine lime juice, oil, parsley, thyme, garlic, and pepper; mix well.

2. Add chicken, yellow squash, and zucchini, tossing to coat. Cover and refrigerate for 2 hours.

3. Alternate chicken, squash, and zucchini onto each of the skewers.

4. Grill 4 inches from heat for 10 minutes, turning frequently. Add cherry tomatoes to each skewer during the last 1 minute of cooking. Remove from heat and serve.

NUTRITION FACTS
4 Servings
Serving Size 3 oz chicken

AMOUNT PER SERVING

Exchanges
1 Vegetable
3 Lean Meat

Calories	189
Calories from Fat	59
Total Fat	7 g
Saturated Fat	1 g
Cholesterol	72 mg
Sodium	67 mg
Total Carbohydrate	4 g
Dietary Fiber	1 g
Sugars	2 g
Protein	27 g

Turkey Burgers

When you tire of the same old hamburgers,
try these for a nice change.

1 1/4 lb ground turkey breast
1/4 cup egg substitute
1/4 tsp onion powder
1/4 tsp dried thyme
1/2 tsp poultry seasoning

1/4 tsp dried sage
Fresh ground pepper (optional)
6 Tbsp Homemade Seasoned Bread
   Crumbs (see recipe, page 223)

1. In a medium bowl, combine all the ingredients except bread crumbs. Scoop meat into 6 patties and press each one lightly into the bread crumbs.

2. Prepare an outside grill or oven broiler and grill or broil 6 inches from heat for 4 to 5 minutes per side until cooked through. Serve warm on split buns and with your favorite condiments.

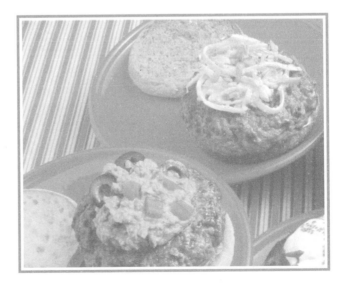

Turkey Cutlets Diane

The classic recipe is made with steak, but this low-fat turkey version is much healthier for you.

2 5-oz boneless, skinless turkey breast cutlets
1 Tbsp flour
Dash salt (optional)
Fresh ground pepper
2 Tbsp reduced-fat margarine (divided use)

1 tsp Dijon mustard
6 large mushrooms, sliced
2 medium scallions, sliced
2 tsp Worcestershire sauce
1 Tbsp cognac
1/2 cup low-sodium chicken broth
2 Tbsp chopped parsley

1. Lightly coat cutlets with a mixture of flour, salt, and pepper. In a large nonstick skillet, melt 1 Tbsp margarine over medium heat.

2. Brown cutlets about 1 to 2 minutes on each side; transfer to a platter. Spread cutlets on both sides with mustard; set aside.

3. Melt remaining margarine in the skillet and sauté mushrooms and scallions over medium heat. Add Worcestershire sauce and cognac and ignite with a long match. Let the flames subside, then add chicken broth.

4. Return cutlets to the skillet; cook until turkey is no longer pink, turning only once. Remove from heat, transfer to a platter, garnish with parsley, and serve.

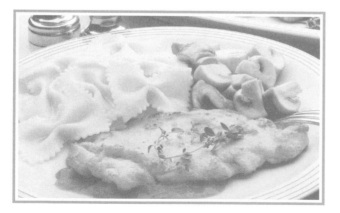

NUTRITION FACTS
2 Servings
Serving Size one cutlet

AMOUNT PER SERVING

Exchanges
1/2 Carbohydrate
5 Very Lean Meat
1 1/2 Fat

Calories	288
Calories from Fat	87
Total Fat	10 g
Saturated Fat	1 g
Cholesterol	93 mg
Sodium	313 mg
Total Carbohydrate	9 g
Dietary Fiber	1 g
Sugars	3 g
Protein	37 g

NUTRITION FACTS

8 Servings
Serving Size 1/8 recipe

AMOUNT PER SERVING

Exchanges
1/2 Carbohydrate
4 Very Lean Meat
1 1/2 Fat

Calories	243	
Calories from Fat	87	
Total Fat	10	g
Saturated Fat	2	g
Cholesterol	80	mg
Sodium	63	mg
Total Carbohydrate	7	g
Dietary Fiber	2	g
Sugars	2	g
Protein	31	g

Turkey with Almond Duxelles

Tucked away inside these moist turkey cutlets is a surprising, crunchy filling of almonds, mushrooms, and shallots.

2 Tbsp olive oil
1/4 cup dry sherry
3/4 lb diced fresh mushrooms
4 medium shallots, finely minced
2 garlic cloves, minced
1 tsp minced fresh thyme
Dash cayenne pepper

1/2 cup ground almonds
Dash salt and pepper
2 lb turkey breast cutlets,
    pounded to 1/4-inch thickness
    and cut into 8 portions
Paprika
1/2 cup reduced-fat sour cream

1. In a large skillet over medium heat, heat the olive oil and sherry. Add the mushrooms, shallots, garlic, thyme, and cayenne pepper. Cook, stirring often, until mushrooms turn dark.

2. Add the ground almonds, salt, and pepper and sauté for 2 to 3 minutes. Divide the mixture into 8 portions and place each portion in the center of each turkey portion. Fold edges over, roll up, and place in a baking dish, seam side down, 1 inch apart.

3. Place about 1 Tbsp of sour cream over each turkey roll and sprinkle with paprika. Bake at 350 degrees for 25 to 30 minutes or until the turkey is tender. Transfer to a serving platter and serve.

Beef, Pork, & Lamb

Apple Cinnamon Pork Chops, 133

Baked Steak with Creole Sauce, 134

Beef Provençal, 135

Beef Shish Kabobs, 136

Butterflied Beef Eye Roast, 137

Herbed Pot Roast, 138

Italian Pork Chops, 139

Lamb Chops with Orange Sauce, 140

Lamb Kabobs, 141

Marinated Beef Kabobs, 142

Marinated Leg of Lamb, 143

Marvelous Meat Loaf, 144

Pork Chops Milanese, 145

Pork Niçoise, 146

Roast Beef with Caraway Seeds, 147

Steak with Brandied Onions, 148

Stir-Fried Pork Tenderloin, 149

Stuffed Bell Peppers, 150

Veal Piccata with Orange Sauce, 151

Veal Romano, 152

Veal Scallopini, 153

NUTRITION FACTS

2 Servings
Serving Size 1 pork chop
with apples

AMOUNT PER SERVING

Exchanges
1 Fruit
2 Lean Meat
1 Fat

Calories	212	
Calories from Fat	92	
Total Fat	10	g
Saturated Fat	2	g
Cholesterol	44	mg
Sodium	36	mg
Total Carbohydrate	15	g
Dietary Fiber	3	g
Sugars	11	g
Protein	16	g

Apple Cinnamon Pork Chops

This dish is great on a crisp fall evening.

2 tsp canola oil
1 large apple, sliced
1/4 tsp cinnamon

1/8 tsp nutmeg
2 3-oz lean boneless pork chops,
   trimmed of fat

1. In a medium nonstick skillet, heat the canola oil. Add apple slices and sauté until just tender. Sprinkle with cinnamon and nutmeg, remove from heat, and keep warm.

2. Place pork chops in skillet and cook thoroughly. Remove pork chops from skillet, arrange on a serving platter, spoon apple slices on top, and serve.

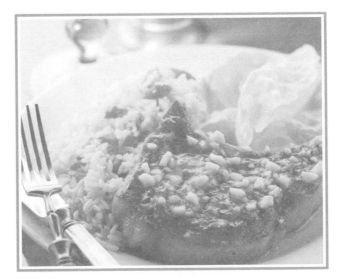

Baked Steak
with Creole Sauce

This spicy creole sauce helps to keep the steak tender and juicy.

2 tsp olive oil
1/4 cup chopped onion
1/4 cup chopped green bell pepper
1 8-oz can crushed tomatoes

1/2 tsp chili powder
1/4 tsp celery seed
1/2 tsp garlic powder
1 lb lean boneless round steak

1. In a large skillet over medium heat, heat the oil. Add the onions and green pepper and sauté until onions are translucent (about 5 minutes).

2. Add the tomatoes and the seasonings; cover and let simmer over low heat for 20 to 25 minutes. This allows the flavors to blend.

3. Preheat the oven to 350 degrees. Trim all visible fat off the steak.

4. In a nonstick pan or a pan that has been sprayed with nonstick cooking spray, lightly brown the steak on each side. Transfer the steak to a 13 × 9 × 2-inch baking dish; pour the sauce over the steak and cover.

5. Bake for 1 1/4 hours or until steak is tender. Remove from oven; slice steak and arrange on a serving platter. Spoon sauce over the steak and serve.

NUTRITION FACTS
4 Servings
Serving Size 3 oz

AMOUNT PER SERVING

Exchanges
1 Vegetable
3 Lean Meat

Calories	194	
Calories from Fat	72	
Total Fat	8	g
Saturated Fat	2	g
Cholesterol	75	mg
Sodium	148	mg
Total Carbohydrate	4	g
Dietary Fiber	1	g
Sugars	3	g
Protein	25	g

Beef Provençal

Fresh zucchini and cherry tomatoes add color to this easy-to-make dish.

3 garlic cloves, minced
1 tsp dried basil
Fresh ground pepper
1 lb lean top sirloin steak, cut into
  4 portions

1 1/2 tsp olive oil
2 small zucchini, thinly sliced
6 cherry tomatoes, halved
2 Tbsp grated fresh Parmesan
  cheese

1. In a small bowl, combine the garlic, basil, and pepper. Divide the mixture in half and rub one half of this mixture on both sides of the steaks. Reserve remaining seasonings.

2. In a large skillet over medium heat, heat the oil. Add the seasonings and heat for 30 seconds. Add the zucchini and sauté for 3 minutes.

3. Add the tomatoes and continue sautéing for 1 to 2 minutes. Remove from heat and transfer to a serving platter, sprinkle with cheese, and keep warm.

4. Add the steaks, 2 at a time, and pan-fry until desired degree of doneness; transfer to a platter and serve them with the vegetables.

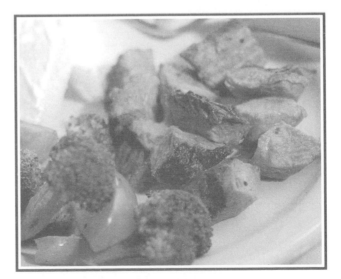

Beef Shish Kabobs

*While the kabobs are cooking, simmer some rice, and
add a salad for a complete meal.*

2 tsp canola oil
1/4 cup red wine vinegar
1 Tbsp lite soy sauce
1 garlic clove, minced
1 Tbsp lemon juice
Fresh ground pepper

1 1/2 lb boneless beef top sirloin
    steak, cut into 24 cubes
2 large bell peppers, red and green,
    cut into 1-inch pieces
1 lb mushrooms, stemmed
1 large tomato, cut into wedges
1 medium onion, quartered

1. Combine the oil, vinegar, soy sauce, garlic, lemon juice, and pepper in a
   small bowl. Pour over the beef cubes and let marinate in the refrigerator
   3 to 4 hours or overnight.

2. Place 3 beef cubes on 8 metal or wooden skewers (remember to soak
   the wooden skewers in water before using), alternating with peppers,
   mushroom caps, tomato wedges, and onions.

3. Grill over medium heat, turning and basting with marinade. Arrange
   skewers on a platter to serve.

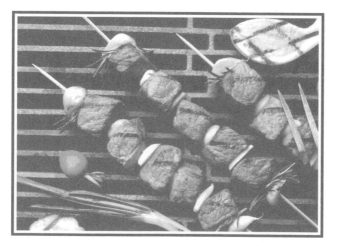

NUTRITION FACTS

8 Servings
Serving Size 1 kabob with
** 2 oz beef plus vegetables**

AMOUNT PER SERVING

Exchanges
2 Vegetable
2 Lean Meat

Calories	42	
Calories from Fat	42	
Total Fat	5	g
Saturated Fat	1	g
Cholesterol	32	mg
Sodium	112	mg
Total Carbohydrate	9	g
Dietary Fiber	2	g
Sugars	4	g
Protein	19	g

Butterflied Beef Eye Roast

Since this is a large piece of meat, be sure to let it marinate overnight or even for two days.

1 3-lb lean beef eye roast
3 Tbsp olive oil
1/4 cup water
1/2 cup red wine vinegar

3 garlic cloves, minced
1/2 tsp crushed red pepper
1 Tbsp chopped fresh thyme

1. Slice the roast down the middle, open it, and lay it flat in a shallow baking dish. In a small bowl, combine the remaining ingredients and pour the mixture over the roast. Cover and let the meat marinate for at least 12 hours. Turn the roast occasionally.

2. Set the oven to broil. Remove the roast from the marinade, discard the marinade, and place the roast on a rack in the broiler pan. Broil the roast 5 to 7 inches from the heat, turning occasionally, for 20 to 25 minutes or until desired degree of doneness.

3. Remove from oven, cover with foil, and let stand for 15 to 20 minutes before carving. Transfer to a serving platter, spoon any juices over the top, and serve.

Herbed Pot Roast

This lean roast simmers slowly in an herb marinade.

1 Tbsp olive oil
1 2-lb lean boneless beef roast
Fresh ground pepper
1/2 cup water
1/3 cup dry sherry
1/4 cup ketchup
1 garlic clove, minced
1/4 tsp dry mustard

1/4 tsp marjoram
1/4 tsp dried rosemary
1/4 tsp dried thyme
2 medium onions, sliced
1 bay leaf
1 16-oz can sliced mushrooms, undrained

1. Add olive oil to a large Dutch oven over medium heat. Sprinkle roast with pepper, then brown roast on all sides.

2. Combine water, sherry, ketchup, garlic, mustard, marjoram, rosemary, and thyme in a small bowl, and pour over roast. Add onions and bay leaf, cover, and simmer for 2 to 3 hours, until roast is tender.

3. Add mushrooms and continue simmering until heated. Remove bay leaf. Transfer roast to a platter, slice, and serve.

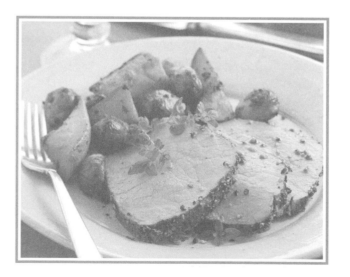

NUTRITION FACTS
8 Servings
Serving Size 3 oz

AMOUNT PER SERVING

Exchanges
1/2 Starch
3 Lean Meat
1/2 Fat

Calories	232
Calories from Fat	82
Total Fat	9 g
Saturated Fat	3 g
Cholesterol	87 mg
Sodium	288 mg
Total Carbohydrate	7 g
Dietary Fiber	1 g
Sugars	3 g
Protein	29 g

Italian Pork Chops

*Serve this with fresh steamed broccoli and
either flavored rice or shaped pasta.*

4 3-oz lean boneless pork chops
Fresh ground pepper
1/2 lb fresh mushrooms, sliced
1 medium onion, chopped
2 garlic cloves, crushed
2 medium green bell peppers,
  julienned
1 8-oz can tomato sauce
1 8-oz can no-salt-added
  tomato sauce
1/4 cup dry sherry
1 Tbsp fresh lemon juice
1/4 tsp dried oregano
1/4 tsp dried basil

1. Trim all excess fat from the pork chops and sprinkle with pepper. Coat a large skillet with nonstick cooking spray, place chops in skillet, and brown on both sides. Remove chops and keep warm.

2. Spray skillet with nonstick cooking spray and add mushrooms, onion, garlic, and green pepper. Sauté over medium heat until the onions are tender, about 5 to 6 minutes.

3. Return the chops to the skillet and stir in the remaining ingredients. Let simmer uncovered for 15 minutes or until meat is tender and cooked through.

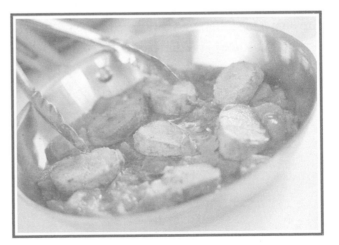

Lamb Chops
with Orange Sauce

*Try serving these delicious orange-scented lamb chops with baby peas
or French green beans.*

1/2 cup unsweetened orange juice
1 Tbsp orange rind
1/2 tsp dried thyme
Fresh ground pepper

8 lean lamb chops, about
  1/2 inch thick
1 Tbsp reduced-fat margarine
1 cup sliced fresh mushrooms
1/2 cup dry white wine

1. In a shallow baking dish, combine the orange juice, orange rind, thyme,
   and pepper; mix well. Trim all excess fat from lamb chops and place in a
   baking dish. Spoon orange juice mixture over chops; cover and refrigerate for 3 to 4 hours, occasionally turning chops.

2. Coat a large skillet with nonstick cooking spray; place over medium-high
   heat until hot. Remove the chops from the marinade, reserving marinade; arrange in the skillet. Brown chops on both sides, remove from
   skillet, and drain.

3. Reduce heat to medium and melt margarine. Add mushrooms and sauté
   until just tender. Stir in reserved marinade and wine and bring to a boil.

4. Return lamb chops to skillet; cover, reduce heat, and simmer for 10 to
   12 minutes or until sauce is reduced to about 1/2 cup. Transfer lamb
   chops to platter, spoon orange sauce on top, and serve.

NUTRITION FACTS

4 Servings
Serving Size 2 lamb chops
  with sauce

AMOUNT PER SERVING

Exchanges
1/2 Starch
3 Lean Meat

Calories	210
Calories from Fat	86
Total Fat	10 g
Saturated Fat	3 g
Cholesterol	72 mg
Sodium	88 mg
Total Carbohydrate	5 g
Dietary Fiber	1 g
Sugars	4 g
Protein	23 g

Lamb Kabobs

These fresh, colorful kabobs are especially good served with wild rice.

1/2 cup low-calorie Italian salad dressing

1/4 cup fresh lemon juice

1 tsp dried oregano

Fresh ground pepper

1 1/2 lb lean boneless lamb, cut into 2-inch pieces

1/2 lb mushrooms, stems removed

10 cherry tomatoes

1 red bell pepper, cut into 1-inch squares

1/2 yellow squash, cut into 1-inch chunks

1. In a shallow baking dish, combine the salad dressing, lemon juice, oregano, and pepper; mix thoroughly. Add lamb; cover, refrigerate, and let marinate for 6 hours or overnight.

2. Remove meat from marinade. Thread the lamb, alternating with vegetables, onto 6 metal or wooden skewers (remember to soak the wooden skewers in water before using). Broil the skewers 7 to 8 inches from the heat for 18 to 20 minutes. Transfer to a platter and serve.

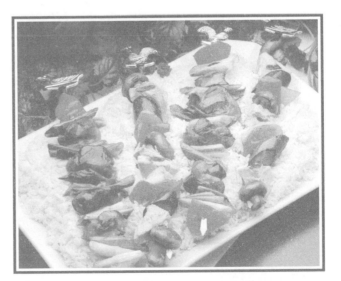

Marinated Beef Kabobs

*The marinade for this dish is quite tasty and easy to prepare.
Try it with chicken, too.*

1 1/2 lb lean sirloin steak, cut into
  1 1/2–inch cubes

1 large red onion, cut into 1-inch
  cubes

1 large green bell pepper, cut into
  1-inch squares

1 large red bell pepper, cut into 1-
  inch squares

1/2 lb mushrooms, stems removed

1/2 cup low-calorie Italian salad
  dressing

1/4 cup burgundy wine

1. Place cubed meat and prepared vegetables together in a shallow dish.
   In a small bowl, combine the salad dressing and wine; blend well. Pour
   the marinade over the meat and vegetables. Cover, refrigerate, and let
   marinate for at least 8 hours, stirring occasionally.

2. Alternate the meat and vegetables on 6 metal or wooden skewers (remember to soak the wooden skewers in water before using).

3. Grill kabobs over medium heat, turning often, for 15 to 20 minutes or
   until desired degree of doneness. Arrange on a platter and serve.

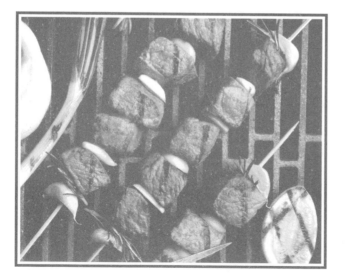

6 Servings
Serving Size 1 kabob

AMOUNT PER SERVING

Exchanges
2 Vegetable
3 Lean Meat

Calories	232
Calories from Fat	75
Total Fat	8 g
Saturated Fat	3 g
Cholesterol	74 mg
Sodium	344 mg
Total Carbohydrate	11 g
Dietary Fiber	2 g
Sugars	5 g
Protein	28 g

Marinated Leg of Lamb

Marinating one to two days is the secret to a great leg of lamb.
Serve with steamed carrots and oven-roasted potatoes.

1 7-lb leg of lamb, boned and
   butterflied
3 cups dry red wine
1/4 cup olive oil
2 medium onions, sliced
1 large carrot, thinly sliced

6 parsley stems
2 bay leaves, crumbled
2 medium cloves garlic, minced
Dash salt (optional)
Fresh ground pepper
Fresh parsley sprigs

1. In a large ceramic, glass, or stainless steel dish (anything but plastic), combine all the ingredients except the parsley sprigs; cover, refrigerate, and let marinate for 1 to 2 days, turning occasionally.

2. After marinating, drain lamb and pat dry. Place lamb into a grill basket. Broil the lamb 3 to 4 inches from the heat for 15 to 20 minutes per side.

3. Transfer lamb to a cutting board and let cool slightly. Carve lamb diagonally; transfer to serving platter, garnish with parsley sprigs and serve.

Marvelous Meat Loaf

*By making meat loaf with beef and turkey, you lower
its fat content significantly.*

1 lb 95% lean ground beef

1 lb ground turkey breast

3/4 cup Homemade Seasoned Bread
Crumbs (see recipe, page 223)

1/2 cup fat-free milk

1/4 cup egg substitute

1 medium onion, finely chopped (for
variety, add 1/4 cup shredded carrot, 2 Tbsp chopped green pepper,
and/or 1/4 cup sliced celery)

1 14.5-oz can stewed tomatoes

1. Preheat the oven to 350 degrees.

2. In a large bowl, combine all ingredients except tomatoes and form into a
   loaf. Place into loaf pan and bake for 1 1/4 to 1 1/2 hours, until internal
   temperature registers 165 degrees. Pour tomatoes over the top during
   the last 20 minutes of baking.

3. Remove from oven, cover with foil, and let stand for 10 minutes before
   serving.

NUTRITION FACTS

10 Servings
Serving Size 3 oz

AMOUNT PER SERVING

Exchanges
1/2 Carbohydrate
2 Very Lean Meat

Calories	105
Calories from Fat	11
Total Fat	1 g
Saturated Fat	1 g
Cholesterol	39 mg
Sodium	198 mg
Total Carbohydrate	8 g
Dietary Fiber	1 g
Sugars	3 g
Protein	16 g

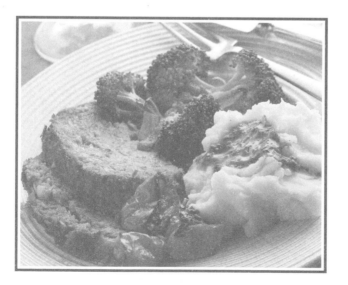

NUTRITION FACTS

4 Servings
Serving Size 1 pork chop

AMOUNT PER SERVING

Exchanges
1 Starch
3 Lean Meat

Calories	246	
Calories from Fat	88	
Total Fat	10	g
Saturated Fat	3	g
Cholesterol	43	mg
Sodium	298	mg
Total Carbohydrate	15	g
Dietary Fiber	1	g
Sugars	2	g
Protein	22	g

Pork Chops Milanese

You will win rave reviews when you prepare these.

1/2 cup Homemade Seasoned Bread
   Crumbs (see recipe, page 223)
1/4 cup fat-free Parmesan cheese
4 3-oz lean boneless pork chops,
   trimmed of fat

1/4 cup flour
1/4 cup egg substitute, slightly
   beaten
2 Tbsp reduced-fat margarine
1 large lemon, cut into wedges

1. Combine bread crumbs and Parmesan cheese in a shallow bowl. Dip
   the pork chops in flour, then egg substitute, and dredge in bread crumb
   mixture.

2. Melt margarine in a large skillet. Add pork chops and brown on both
   sides. Reduce heat, cover, and simmer for 3 to 5 minutes. Remove cover,
   and cook 5 to 10 minutes more until pork is no longer pink.

3. Squeeze 2 or 3 lemon wedges over chops. Transfer to a serving platter,
   garnish with remaining lemon wedges, and serve.

Pork Niçoise

This one-skillet dish is easy to make, but elegant to serve!

1 Tbsp olive oil

18 oz boneless pork tenderloin, trimmed of fat and cut into 6 pieces

4 large tomatoes, chopped

2 garlic cloves, minced

1 large green bell pepper, chopped

1 tsp dried basil

1/2 cup whole black olives

2 cups cooked rice, hot

1. In a large skillet, heat oil over medium heat. Add pork tenderloin and lightly brown on both sides.

2. Add the tomatoes, garlic, green pepper, and basil; cover. Simmer for 25 to 30 minutes, turning pork once. Add the olives and continue to simmer over low heat for 7 to 10 minutes.

3. Arrange rice on serving platter, place tenderloin over rice, spoon sauce over the top, and serve.

NUTRITION FACTS

6 Servings
Serving Size 3 oz pork with topping and 1/3 cup cooked rice

AMOUNT PER SERVING

Exchanges
1 Starch
1 Vegetable
2 Lean Meat

Calories	219
Calories from Fat	55
Total Fat	6 g
Saturated Fat	1 g
Cholesterol	46 mg
Sodium	146 mg
Total Carbohydrate	22 g
Dietary Fiber	3 g
Sugars	4 g
Protein	19 g

Roast Beef with Caraway Seeds

Serve this hearty dish with cabbage and noodles.

3/4 cup chopped onion
1 Tbsp caraway seeds
1 2-lb lean boneless chuck roast
1 Tbsp olive oil

1/3 cup red wine vinegar
1 cup unsweetened apple juice
1 Tbsp minced parsley
1/2 cup water

1. In a small bowl, combine 1/4 cup onion and caraway seeds and press into roast.

2. In a medium saucepan, sauté remaining onion in olive oil. Place roast in a roasting pan and add the sautéd onion.

3. Add vinegar, apple juice, parsley, and water. Bake roast uncovered at 325 degrees for 1 to 1 1/2 hours, basting frequently. Transfer roast to a platter and slice.

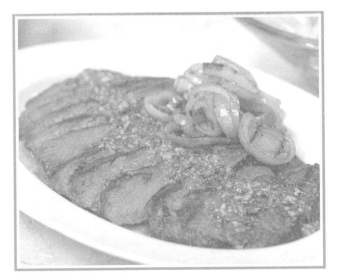

Steak with Brandied Onions

This classic steak is great with a baked potato and a green salad.

12 oz lean sirloin steak
4 Tbsp reduced-fat margarine
1/2 tsp garlic powder

4 medium onions, sliced
1 Tbsp chopped fresh parsley
Dash brandy

1. Prepare the sirloin steak to your liking.
2. In a medium skillet, melt the margarine and add garlic powder. Add the onions and parsley, sautéing until onions are tender.
3. Add brandy and let simmer for 1 to 2 minutes. Transfer steak to platter, spoon brandied onions over the top, and serve.

NUTRITION FACTS

4 Servings
Serving Size 2–3 oz steak
with onions

AMOUNT PER SERVING

Exchanges
2 Vegetable
3 Lean Meat
1/2 Fat

Calories	230
Calories from Fat	102
Total Fat	11 g
Saturated Fat	3 g
Cholesterol	56 mg
Sodium	137 mg
Total Carbohydrate	11 g
Dietary Fiber	2 g
Sugars	7 g
Protein	21 g

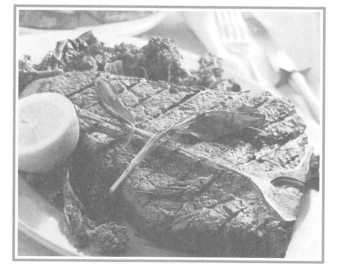

Stir-Fried Pork Tenderloin

The secret to this dish is not to overcook it.

1 lb pork tenderloin, cut into thin strips
1 Tbsp vegetable oil
1 Tbsp oyster sauce (found in the Asian food section of the grocery store)
1 Tbsp cornstarch

1/2 cup low-sodium chicken broth
1 Tbsp lite soy sauce
1 cup fresh snow peas, trimmed
1/2 cup sliced water chestnuts, drained
1/2 cup minced red pepper
1/4 cup sliced scallions

1. In a large skillet or wok, heat oil. Stir-fry pork until strips are no longer pink.
2. Combine oyster sauce, cornstarch, chicken broth, and soy sauce in a measuring cup. Add to the pork and cook until sauce thickens.
3. Add vegetables, cover, and steam for 2 to 3 minutes. Serve.

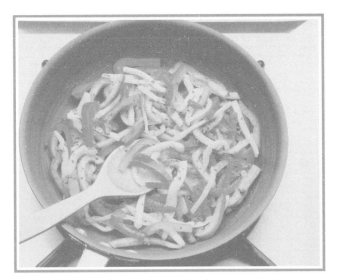

Stuffed Bell Peppers

Try using this basic filling to stuff zucchini or yellow squash, too.

4 medium bell peppers, red or
  green (or both)
1 lb lean ground sirloin
1 small onion, chopped
1/3 cup instant white rice
1 tsp dried oregano

Dash salt
Fresh ground pepper
8 oz canned tomato sauce
1/4 cup burgundy wine
Parmesan cheese to taste (optional)

1. Slice off the stem end of each pepper and remove the seeds. In a medium
   bowl, combine the beef, onion, rice, oregano, salt, pepper, and 1/3 cup
   tomato sauce; mix well.

2. Stuff the mixture into the peppers and place them in a medium saucepan. Pour the wine and remaining tomato sauce over peppers.

3. Bring the peppers to a boil; cover and let simmer until they are tender,
   about 45 minutes. Add a few tablespoons of water if the sauce begins to
   cook away. Transfer to a serving platter, top with Parmesan cheese, and
   serve.

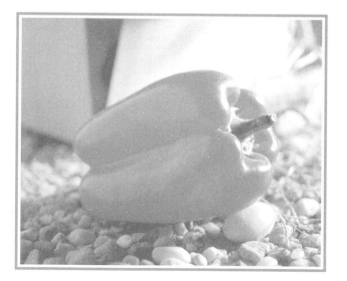

NUTRITION FACTS
4 Servings
Serving Size 1 pepper

AMOUNT PER SERVING

Exchanges
1/2 Starch
2 Vegetable
3 Lean Meat

Calories	251	
Calories from Fat	54	
Total Fat	6	g
Saturated Fat	2	g
Cholesterol	71	mg
Sodium	469	mg
Total Carbohydrate	21	g
Dietary Fiber	2	g
Sugars	6	g
Protein	28	g

NUTRITION FACTS

4 Servings
Serving Size 3–4 oz

AMOUNT PER SERVING

Exchanges
1 Starch
4 Lean Meat

Calories	320
Calories from Fat	106
Total Fat	12 g
Saturated Fat	3 g
Cholesterol	117 mg
Sodium	204 mg
Total Carbohydrate	18 g
Dietary Fiber	1 g
Sugars	8 g
Protein	34 g

Veal Piccata with Orange Sauce

Fresh orange juice and sage make all the difference in this recipe—but they do need to be fresh!

1/2 cup flour
Dash salt and pepper
6 Tbsp reduced-fat margarine
1 lb lean veal cutlets

1 cup fresh orange juice
1 tsp minced fresh sage
1 orange, sliced
1 Tbsp minced fresh parsley

1. Place flour on a large plate and season with pepper and salt. In a large skillet, melt 4 Tbsp of margarine. Coat the veal with flour, shaking off excess. Add to the skillet, in batches, and cook for 30 seconds on each side. Transfer to a warm plate and keep warm.

2. Discard the pan drippings. Add 1/2 cup of the orange juice to the pan and bring to a boil, scraping up any browned bits. Boil for 1 to 2 minutes or until juice is reduced to a glaze.

3. Add remaining 1/2 cup orange juice and sage; season with salt and pepper and bring back to a boil. Boil for 1 to 2 minutes or until mixture thickens.

4. Remove from heat and whisk in remaining 2 Tbsp of margarine. Transfer veal to a platter, spoon orange sauce on top, and garnish with orange slices and fresh parsley to serve.

Veal Romano

You can buy the roasted peppers for this dish in the condiment aisle of the supermarket (they come in jars), or in a gourmet deli.

2 Tbsp olive oil
1 1/2 lb lean veal cutlets
1/4 cup flour
Fresh ground pepper
2 Tbsp reduced-fat margarine

1/2 cup dry white wine
1/2 cup roasted red peppers,
  drained and julienned
8 large black olives, thinly sliced
2 Tbsp capers, rinsed and drained

1. Heat the oil in a skillet over high heat. Place the cutlets between two pieces of waxed paper and pound with a meat mallet until they are about 1/4 inch thick.

2. Lightly flour the veal, shaking off the excess, and add to the skillet. Sauté the veal for 2 to 3 minutes on each side, transfer to a platter, and sprinkle with pepper. Continue until all veal is cooked.

3. Melt the margarine in the skillet over high heat. Add the wine and scrape the brown bits from the skillet. Reduce heat to medium and add the red peppers, olives, and capers, stirring occasionally.

4. Continue cooking until heated through. Spoon the sauce over the veal and serve.

NUTRITION FACTS

6 Servings
Serving Size 3–4 oz

AMOUNT PER SERVING

Exchanges
1/2 Starch
4 Lean Meat

Calories	270	
Calories from Fat	106	
Total Fat	12	g
Saturated Fat	3	g
Cholesterol	117	mg
Sodium	189	mg
Total Carbohydrate	5	g
Dietary Fiber	1	g
Sugars	1	g
Protein	33	g

Veal Scallopini

*Serve this classic dish with vermicelli and
steamed broccoli or green beans.*

4 lean veal cutlets (3–4 oz each)
Fresh ground pepper
1 Tbsp olive oil
1/2 lb fresh mushrooms, sliced
1 large green bell pepper, cut into
   1/2-inch strips

1/2 cup dry white wine
1/3 cup low-sodium chicken broth
1 Tbsp lemon juice
1 Tbsp cornstarch
2 Tbsp water
2 Tbsp minced fresh parsley

1. Place the veal cutlets between two pieces of waxed paper and pound until the cutlets are 1/8 inch thick. Sprinkle the veal with pepper and set aside.

2. Over medium heat, heat the oil in a large skillet. Add the veal, a few pieces at a time, cooking 2 to 3 minutes per side or until lightly browned. Remove from skillet and keep the veal warm while you prepare the sauce.

3. Sauté the mushrooms and green pepper in the skillet for 3 minutes. Add the wine, broth, and lemon juice and bring to a boil. Dissolve the cornstarch with the water and add to the skillet, stirring constantly until mixture has thickened.

4. Remove from heat and stir in the parsley. Arrange the veal on a serving platter and pour the sauce over the top.

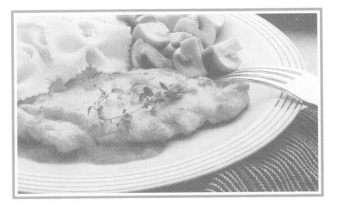

Seafood

Baked Fish in Foil, 157

Baked Garlic Scampi, 158

Baked Shrimp, 159

Baked Shrimp and Mushroom Casserole, 160

Basic Boiled Shrimp, 161

Broiled Sole with Mustard Sauce, 162

Crab Imperial, 163

Crabmeat Stuffing, 164

Fish Fillets with Tomatoes, 165

Flounder Parmesan, 166

Fresh Flounder Creole, 167

Grilled Salmon with Dill Sauce, 168

Grilled Scallop Kabobs, 169

Grilled Shark, 170

Grilled Swordfish with Rosemary, 171

Halibut Supreme, 172

Lobster Fricassee, 173

Pan-Fried Scallops, 174

Poached Red Snapper, 175

Sea Bass with Ginger Sauce, 176

Shrimp Creole, 177

Shrimp Provençal, 178

Trout Amandine, 179

Vegetable Salmon Cakes, 180

Baked Fish in Foil

Preparing fish in foil is an easy and flavorful cooking method.

1 3-lb whole red snapper or bass, cleaned
1 medium garlic clove, minced
1/4 cup olive oil
Fresh ground pepper
1/2 tsp dried thyme
1 tsp flour

1/2 lb large shrimp, shelled and deveined
1/2 lb sliced mushrooms
3 Tbsp lemon juice
1/2 cup dry white wine
1/4 cup minced parsley
1 tsp grated lemon peel

1. Wash fish, inside and out, under cold running water, and pat dry with paper towels.
2. In a small bowl, combine garlic, olive oil, pepper, thyme, and flour and mix well.
3. Place fish on a double thickness of heavy aluminum foil. In the cavity of the fish, place 1 Tbsp garlic mixture, 4 shrimp, and 1/2 cup sliced mushrooms. Sprinkle with 1 Tbsp lemon juice and 2 Tbsp wine.
4. Dot top of fish with remaining garlic mixture and arrange remaining shrimp and mushrooms on top. Sprinkle with remaining lemon juice and wine, parsley, and lemon peel.
5. Bring the long sides of the foil together over the fish and secure with a double fold. Fold both ends of foil upward several times.
6. Place fish on a cookie sheet; bake at 375 degrees for 30 to 35 minutes. Transfer to a serving platter and serve.

Baked Garlic Scampi

Scampi is always delicious served over a bed of rice. Remember to buy one pound of shrimp, total weight (with shells on).

1/3 cup reduced-fat margarine
Dash salt
7 garlic cloves, crushed
2 Tbsp chopped parsley

1 lb large shrimp, shelled, deveined, with tails left on
1 tsp grated lemon peel
1 Tbsp lemon juice

1. In a 13 × 9 × 2-inch baking pan, melt the margarine in a 400-degree oven. Add the salt, garlic, and 1 Tbsp parsley; mix well.
2. Arrange the shrimp in a single layer in the baking pan and bake at 350 degrees for 3 minutes, uncovered. Turn the shrimp and sprinkle with lemon peel, lemon juice, and the remaining 1 Tbsp parsley. Continue to bake 1 to 2 minutes more until the shrimp are bright pink and tender.
3. Remove shrimp from oven and arrange on a warm serving platter. Spoon garlic mixture over shrimp and serve.

NUTRITION FACTS
4 Servings
Serving Size 3 oz

AMOUNT PER SERVING

Exchanges
3 Lean Meat

Calories	166
Calories from Fat	76
Total Fat	8 g
Saturated Fat	2 g
Cholesterol	180 mg
Sodium	331 mg
Total Carbohydrate	2 g
Dietary Fiber	0 g
Sugars	2 g
Protein	20 g

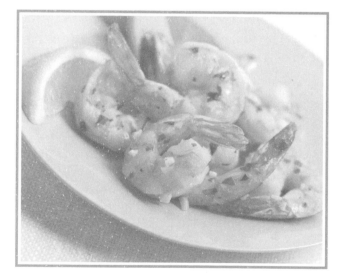

Baked Shrimp

Although great for every day, don't hesitate
to prepare this for guests, too.

16 raw large shrimp

2 Tbsp olive oil

1–2 Tbsp water

1/2 cup chopped parsley

3 garlic cloves, minced

1 cup dried bread crumbs

2 tsp paprika

1 large lemon, cut into wedges

1. With a small knife, cut down the back of the shrimp, but not all the way through, and flatten slightly. Place shrimp in a baking dish.

2. Combine olive oil, water, parsley, garlic, bread crumbs, and paprika. Mix thoroughly and spoon mixture on each shrimp. Bake for 10 minutes at 400 degrees and garnish with lemon wedges.

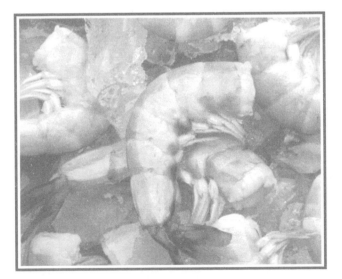

Baked Shrimp and Mushroom Casserole

These tender shrimp are covered with a light sherry cream sauce. Remember to buy two pounds of shrimp, total weight (with shells on).

2 Tbsp canola oil

2 Tbsp reduced-fat margarine

1 lb mushrooms, sliced

2 Tbsp flour

1 tsp salt

Fresh ground pepper

1/8 tsp nutmeg

1 cup fat-free half-and-half

2 lb shrimp, shelled, deveined, and boiled for 2 minutes

1/2 cup dry sherry

1/2 cup Homemade Seasoned Bread Crumbs (see recipe, page 223)

2 Tbsp chopped almonds

1 Tbsp chopped parsley

1. Preheat the oven to 350 degrees.

2. In a large nonstick skillet over medium heat, heat the oil. Add the mushrooms and sauté for 3 to 5 minutes. With a slotted spoon, remove the mushrooms and arrange on the bottom of a 1 1/2–quart baking dish.

3. Melt the margarine in the skillet. Whisk in flour, salt, pepper, and nutmeg until smooth. Gradually add the half-and-half and bring to a boil, stirring constantly. Reduce heat and simmer until thickened.

4. Add the shrimp and sherry, mixing well. Spoon the shrimp mixture over the mushrooms in the baking dish. Mix the bread crumbs and almonds; sprinkle over the shrimp and top with parsley.

5. Bake uncovered for 20 minutes or until the casserole is heated through and bubbly. Remove from the oven and serve hot.

NUTRITION FACTS
8 Servings
Serving Size 2 1/2–3 oz

AMOUNT PER SERVING

Exchanges
1/2 Carbohydrate
2 Very Lean Meat
1 1/2 Fat

Calories 190
Calories from Fat 73
Total Fat 8 g
Saturated Fat 1 g
Cholesterol 133 mg
Sodium 537 mg
Total Carbohydrate 10 g
Dietary Fiber 1 g
Sugars 3 g
Protein 17 g

Basic Boiled Shrimp

This is a good basic recipe to prepare shrimp for cocktail sauce.

4 bay leaves
20 peppercorns
12 whole cloves
1 tsp cayenne pepper
1 tsp dried marjoram
1/2 tsp dried basil
1/4 tsp dried thyme
1/8 tsp caraway seeds

1 tsp mustard seeds
1/8 tsp cumin seeds
1/4 tsp fennel seeds
8 cups water
1 large lemon, quartered
1 garlic clove, minced
2 lb large shrimp, shelled and deveined

1. In a double or triple thickness of cheesecloth, combine all the spices (first 11 ingredients). Secure the packet with a piece of string.

2. Combine water, lemon, garlic, and spice bag together in a Dutch oven. Bring the water to a boil, reduce the heat, and simmer for 3 minutes.

3. Add shrimp and return to a boil. Boil shrimp for 3 to 5 minutes. Drain thoroughly and chill. Serve with cocktail sauce.

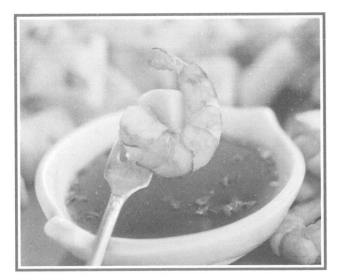

Broiled Sole with Mustard Sauce

This delicious sauce keeps fish moist.
Try it over cooked broccoli or string beans, too.

1 1/2 lb fresh sole fillets

3 Tbsp low-fat mayonnaise

2 Tbsp Dijon mustard

1 Tbsp chopped parsley

Fresh ground pepper

1 large lemon, cut into wedges

1. Coat a baking sheet with nonstick cooking spray. Arrange fillets so they don't overlap.

2. In a small bowl, combine the mayonnaise, mustard, parsley, and pepper and mix thoroughly. Spread the mixture evenly over the fillets. Broil 3 to 4 inches from the heat for 4 minutes until fish flakes easily with a fork.

3. Arrange fillets on a serving platter, garnish with lemon wedges, and serve.

NUTRITION FACTS

6 Servings
Serving Size 3 oz with sauce

AMOUNT PER SERVING

Exchanges
2 Lean Meat

Calories	129	
Calories from Fat	34	
Total Fat	4	g
Saturated Fat	1	g
Cholesterol	63	mg
Sodium	201	mg
Total Carbohydrate	1	g
Dietary Fiber	0	g
Sugars	1	g
Protein	22	g

NUTRITION FACTS

6 Servings
Serving Size 3 oz
 (1 custard cup)

AMOUNT PER SERVING

Exchanges
2 Medium-Fat Meat

Calories	143
Calories from Fat	72
Total Fat	8 g
Saturated Fat	2 g
Cholesterol	75 mg
Sodium	361 mg
Total Carbohydrate	2 g
Dietary Fiber	0 g
Sugars	1 g
Protein	15 g

Crab Imperial

*This dish is suitable to serve as a light party luncheon entree
or as an appetizer for dinner.*

1 lb canned crabmeat, rinsed,
 drained, and flaked
1/4 cup egg substitute, slightly
 beaten
1/2 cup low-fat mayonnaise

2 Tbsp fat-free milk
2 tsp capers
Fresh ground pepper
3 Tbsp Parmesan cheese
1/4 cup chopped parsley

1. Preheat the oven to 350 degrees. In a medium bowl, combine the crabmeat, egg substitute, mayonnaise, milk, capers, and pepper. Stir until
 well blended.

2. Coat 6 custard cups with nonstick cooking spray and divide the mixture
 evenly into the cups. Sprinkle the tops with cheese and bake for 25 to 30
 minutes.

3. Remove from the oven and garnish with chopped parsley before serving.

Crabmeat Stuffing

Use this stuffing to fill the cavity of a zucchini or yellow squash.

1/4 cup reduced-fat margarine
1/4 cup flour
1 cup fat-free milk
1/2 Tbsp Worcestershire sauce
2 lb canned crabmeat, rinsed,
  drained, and flaked

1/4 tsp nutmeg
1 Tbsp chopped red bell pepper
2 Tbsp minced parsley
Dash salt
Fresh ground pepper

1. Melt the margarine in a large skillet over medium heat; add flour and whisk until smooth.

2. Add the milk; continue cooking, stirring constantly, until thickened.

3. Add remaining ingredients; mix thoroughly. Continue to cook until crabmeat is heated through.

NUTRITION FACTS
8 Servings
Serving Size 4 oz

AMOUNT PER SERVING

Exchanges
1/2 Starch
2 Lean Meat

Calories	150	
Calories from Fat	41	
Total Fat	5	g
Saturated Fat	1	g
Cholesterol	97	mg
Sodium	357	mg
Total Carbohydrate	5	g
Dietary Fiber	0	g
Sugars	21	g
Protein	21	g

Fish Fillets with Tomatoes

Use any white fish you like. This recipe is good with orange roughy, flounder, sole, or perch.

1 medium tomato, minced
1 Tbsp minced onion
1/2 tsp fresh dill
1/4 tsp dried basil
1 lb fish fillets

2 Tbsp olive oil
1 Tbsp lemon juice
1/4 cup water
1 lemon, cut into wedges

1. Combine tomato, onion, dill, and basil.

2. Place fillets in a skillet and brush with the olive oil. Spoon tomato mixture over fish. Add lemon juice and water.

3. Simmer fillets over medium heat for 8 to 10 minutes. Transfer to a serving platter and garnish with lemon wedges.

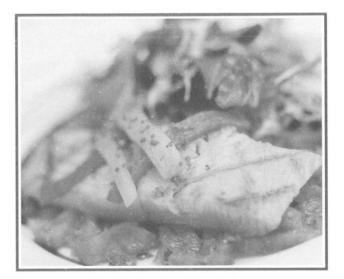

Flounder Parmesan

Instead of frying, why not have light baked fish?

4 4-oz flounder fillets

1/4 cup fresh grated Parmesan
  cheese

1 tsp dried oregano

1/4 tsp dried basil

1 Tbsp minced onion

1 tsp garlic powder

2 tsp paprika

2 Tbsp finely minced parsley

Fresh ground pepper

8 oz fat-free sour cream

1. Place fish fillets in a baking dish.

2. Combine the remaining ingredients and spread over fish. Bake for 12 to
   15 minutes at 375 degrees. Transfer to a platter and serve.

NUTRITION FACTS

4 Servings
Serving Size 3–4 oz

AMOUNT PER SERVING

Exchanges
1/2 Starch
4 Very Lean Meat

Calories	184	
Calories from Fat	30	
Total Fat	3	g
Saturated Fat	1	g
Cholesterol	71	mg
Sodium	172	mg
Total Carbohydrate	4	g
Dietary Fiber	0	g
Sugars	3	g
Protein	28	g

NUTRITION FACTS

4 Servings
Serving Size 3 oz fish

AMOUNT PER SERVING

Exchanges
2 Vegetable
2 Lean Meat

Calories	155	
Calories from Fat	30	
Total Fat	3	g
Saturated Fat	1	g
Cholesterol	59	mg
Sodium	102	mg
Total Carbohydrate	9	g
Dietary Fiber	2	g
Sugars	6	g
Protein	23	g

Fresh Flounder Creole

Add a touch of New Orleans to dinner!

1 lb flounder fillets
3/4 cup chopped tomato
1/4 cup chopped green bell pepper
3 Tbsp fresh lemon juice
1 1/2 tsp olive oil
2 tsp hot pepper sauce

1 tsp finely chopped onion
1/2 tsp dried basil
1/2 tsp celery seed
1 large green bell pepper, sliced
   into rings
1 tomato, cut into wedges

1. Preheat the oven to 400 degrees. Spray a 13 × 9 × 2-inch baking dish with nonstick cooking spray; place fillets in the dish. In a medium bowl, combine all the ingredients except for the garnish; mix thoroughly.

2. Spoon creole mixture over fillets and bake for 10 minutes or until fish flakes easily with a fork. Transfer to a platter and garnish with pepper rings and tomato wedges to serve.

Grilled Salmon with Dill Sauce

Moisten these grilled salmon steaks with plain yogurt perked up with dill.

1 cup plain fat-free yogurt
2 tsp minced fresh dill
1/4 cup chopped scallions
1 tsp capers

2 tsp minced parsley
1 tsp minced chives
1 Tbsp olive oil
2 lb salmon steaks

1. In a small bowl, combine the first six ingredients and set aside. Spray the racks of your grill with nonstick cooking spray.

2. Brush the salmon steaks with olive oil and grill them over medium-hot coals for 4 minutes per side, or just until the salmon flakes with a fork.

3. Transfer the salmon to a platter and serve with dill sauce on the side.

NUTRITION FACTS

8 Servings
Serving Size 3–4 oz salmon
  with 2 Tbsp sauce

AMOUNT PER SERVING

Exchanges
4 Lean Meat

Calories	218	
Calories from Fat	103	
Total Fat	11	g
Saturated Fat	2	g
Cholesterol	79	mg
Sodium	81	mg
Total Carbohydrate	2	g
Dietary Fiber	0	g
Sugars	2	g
Protein	26	g

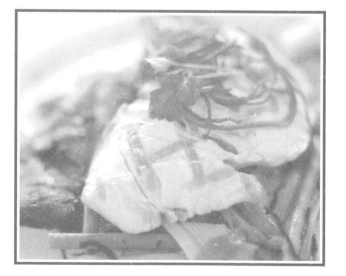

Grilled Scallop Kabobs

Your guests will have fun preparing their own kabobs.

15 oz pineapple chunks, packed in their own juice, undrained
1/4 cup dry white wine
1/4 cup lite soy sauce
2 Tbsp minced parsley
1 tsp minced garlic
Fresh ground pepper
1 lb scallops
18 large cherry tomatoes
1 large green bell pepper, cut into 1-inch squares
18 medium mushroom caps

1. Drain the pineapple, reserving the juice. In a shallow baking dish, combine the pineapple juice, wine, soy sauce, parsley, garlic, and pepper. Mix well.
2. Add the pineapple, scallops, tomatoes, green pepper, and mushrooms. Marinate 30 minutes at room temperature, stirring occasionally.
3. Alternate pineapple, scallops, and vegetables on metal or wooden skewers (remember to soak the wooden skewers in water before using).
4. Grill the kabobs over medium-hot coals about 4 to 5 inches from the heat, turning frequently, for 5 to 7 minutes.

Grilled Shark

This recipe brings out the natural flavor in shark without a lot of complicated ingredients.

1 lb shark fillets
3 Tbsp fresh lime juice
Fresh ground pepper
2 tsp olive oil

1 Tbsp fresh chopped mint
1 Tbsp fresh chopped cilantro
1 garlic clove, minced

1. Wash the shark fillets and combine with the lime juice. Sprinkle with pepper. Marinate refrigerated for 1 to 2 hours.

2. Combine oil, mint, cilantro, and garlic. Brush fillets with mixture. Grill over medium heat for 6 to 8 minutes, turning once. Transfer to a platter and serve.

NUTRITION FACTS

4 Servings
Serving Size 3 oz

AMOUNT PER SERVING

Exchanges
3 Lean Meat

Calories	161
Calories from Fat	62
Total Fat	7 g
Saturated Fat	2 g
Cholesterol	44 mg
Sodium	103 mg
Total Carbohydrates	1 g
Dietary Fiber	0 g
Sugars	1 g
Protein	23 g

4 Servings
Serving Size 3 oz

AMOUNT PER SERVING

Exchanges
3 Lean Meat
1/2 Fat

Calories	199
Calories from Fat	102
Total Fat	11 g
Saturated Fat	2 g
Cholesterol	44 mg
Sodium	102 mg
Total Carbohydrate	1 g
Dietary Fiber	0 g
Sugars	1 g
Protein	22 g

Grilled Swordfish with Rosemary

When preparing swordfish, no need to fuss. Just a few touches here and there produces wonderful fish.

2 scallions, thinly sliced
2 Tbsp olive oil
2 Tbsp white wine vinegar

1 tsp fresh rosemary
4 swordfish steaks (3–4 oz each)

1. Combine the marinade ingredients and pour over the swordfish steaks. Let marinate for 30 minutes.

2. Remove steaks from marinade, and grill for 5 to 7 minutes per side, brushing with marinade. Transfer to a serving platter and serve.

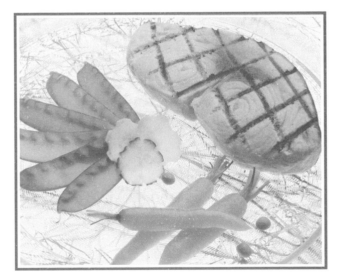

Halibut Supreme

This halibut has a crunchy almond topping.

1 1/2 lb halibut steaks	3/4 cup water
1 cup sliced mushrooms	Dash salt
1 Tbsp olive oil	Fresh ground pepper
1 small onion, finely chopped	1/4 cup toasted almond slivers
3 Tbsp white wine	1 Tbsp chopped parsley

1. Coat a 13 × 9 × 2-inch baking dish with cooking spray, and place halibut steaks in baking dish.
2. Add the remaining ingredients, except almonds and parsley, and bake at 325 degrees, basting frequently, for 25 minutes until fish flakes easily with a fork.
3. Remove from oven and top the halibut steaks with toasted almond slivers. Garnish with parsley.

NUTRITION FACTS

6 Servings
Serving Size 3 oz

AMOUNT PER SERVING

Exchanges
1 Vegetable
3 Lean Meat

Calories	186
Calories from Fat	66
Total Fat	7 g
Saturated Fat	1 g
Cholesterol	37 mg
Sodium	85 mg
Total Carbohydrate	3 g
Dietary Fiber	1 g
Sugars	2 g
Protein	25 g

Lobster Fricassee

*A fricassee is traditionally served in a white sauce,
but this low-fat version tastes just as good!*

2 cups shelled lobster meat
1/4 cup low-fat margarine
3/4 lb mushrooms, sliced
1/2 tsp onion powder
1/2 cup fat-free milk

1/4 cup flour
1/4 tsp paprika
Dash salt and pepper
2 cups cooked rice or pasta
Parsley sprigs

1. Cut the lobster meat into bite-sized pieces. Melt the margarine in a saucepan; add the mushrooms and onion powder. Sauté for 5 to 6 minutes.

2. Whisk the milk and flour in a small bowl, whisking quickly to eliminate any lumps. Pour milk mixture into mushroom mixture; mix thoroughly, and continue cooking for 3 to 5 minutes.

3. Add the lobster, paprika, salt, and pepper; continue cooking for 5 to 10 minutes until lobster is heated through.

4. Spread rice or pasta onto a serving platter, spoon lobster and sauce over the top, and garnish with parsley to serve.

Pan-Fried Scallops

Some people think scallops taste best when they are lightly pan-fried, which seals in all the natural juices.

1/2 cup dried bread crumbs
1/4 tsp paprika
Dash salt and pepper
1 1/2 lb scallops

1/4 cup olive oil
1 Tbsp reduced-fat margarine
2 cups cooked rice, hot
1/4 cup dry white wine

1. Combine the bread crumbs, paprika, salt, and pepper in a small bowl. Roll the scallops thoroughly in the bread crumb mixture.

2. In a large skillet, heat the olive oil and margarine and sauté the scallops quickly for about 2 to 3 minutes until lightly browned.

3. Spread the hot cooked rice on a serving platter and gently place the cooked scallops on top of the rice. Add the white wine to the remaining olive oil–margarine mixture in the pan. Bring to a slow boil. Remove from heat and pour over the rice and scallops to serve.

NUTRITION FACTS

6 Servings
Serving Size 3–4 oz with
 1/3 cup rice

AMOUNT PER SERVING

Exchanges
1 1/2 Starch
2 Medium-Fat Meat

Calories	280
Calories from Fat	104
Total Fat	12 g
Saturated Fat	2 g
Cholesterol	39 mg
Sodium	312 mg
Total Carbohydrate	22 g
Dietary Fiber	1 g
Sugars	1 g
Protein	20 g

Poached Red Snapper

The whole fish is presented in this recipe. Have your fish market clean and scale the fish for you, but do leave on the head and tail.

1 cup dry white wine

1 medium lemon, sliced

6 parsley sprigs

5 peppercorns

5 scallions, sliced

2 bay leaves

1/2 tsp salt (optional)

1/2–1 cup water

1 pan-dressed red snapper
(about 1 1/2–2 lb)

1 lemon, sliced

Parsley sprigs

1. In a fish poacher or very large skillet, combine the wine, lemon slices, parsley sprigs, peppercorns, scallions, bay leaves, salt, and water. Bring the mixture to a boil; add the snapper.

2. Cover the pan, lower the heat, and simmer the red snapper for 15 to 20 minutes until the fish flakes easily with a fork.

3. Carefully lift out the snapper and transfer to a platter. Garnish with lemon slices and parsley.

Sea Bass
with Ginger Sauce

*Steaming fish is the healthiest way to prepare it—
and it's always moist, never dried out.*

2 4-oz sea bass fillets

1 Tbsp canola oil

2 Tbsp minced fresh ginger

2 garlic cloves, minced

1/3 cup minced scallions

4 tsp chopped cilantro

2 Tbsp lite soy sauce

1. In a medium steamer, add water and bring to a boil. Arrange the fillets on the steamer rack. Cover and steam for 6 to 8 minutes.

2. Meanwhile, heat the oil in a small skillet. Add the ginger and garlic and sauté for 2 to 3 minutes.

3. Transfer the steamed fillets to a platter. Pour ginger oil over the fillets and top with scallions, cilantro, and soy sauce.

NUTRITION FACTS

2 Servings
Serving Size 3–4 oz

AMOUNT PER SERVING

Exchanges
1 Vegetable
3 Lean Meat

Calories	198	
Calories from Fat	84	
Total Fat	9	g
Saturated Fat	1	g
Cholesterol	47	mg
Sodium	655	mg
Total Carbohydrate	5	g
Dietary Fiber	1	g
Sugars	2	g
Protein	23	g

Shrimp Creole

NUTRITION FACTS

4 Servings
Serving Size 2–3 oz shrimp
with 1/2 cup cooked rice

AMOUNT PER SERVING

Exchanges
2 Starch
1 Lean Meat

Calories	213	
Calories from Fat	10	
Total Fat	1	g
Saturated Fat	0	g
Cholesterol	131	mg
Sodium	534	mg
Total Carbohydrate	31	g
Dietary Fiber	2	g
Sugars	4	g
Protein	18	g

*This creole sauce is really versatile—you can add chicken cubes,
lobster chunks, mussels, or clams instead of shrimp.
Remember to buy one pound of shrimp,
total weight (with shells on).*

1 8-oz can tomato sauce
1/2 cup sliced mushrooms
1/2 cup dry white wine
1/2 cup chopped onion
2 garlic cloves, minced
1/2 cup chopped green bell pepper

1/2 cup chopped celery
2 bay leaves
1/4 tsp cayenne pepper
1 lb shrimp, shelled and deveined
2 cups cooked rice, hot

1. In a large skillet, combine the tomato sauce, mushrooms, wine, onion, garlic, green pepper, celery, bay leaves, and cayenne pepper. Bring to a boil; cover, reduce the heat, and let simmer for 10 to 15 minutes.

2. Add the shrimp to the tomato sauce and cook uncovered for 3 to 5 minutes, until the shrimp are bright pink.

3. To serve, spread the rice on a platter, and spoon the shrimp and creole sauce over the rice.

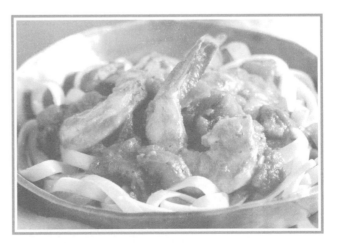

Shrimp Provençal

Serve crusty French bread to soak up this warm shallot and tomato sauce. Remember to buy two pounds of shrimp, total weight (with shells on).

2 Tbsp olive oil
1/4 cup chopped shallots
1 garlic clove, crushed
1 tomato, peeled and coarsely
   chopped
8 oz tomato sauce
Dash salt and pepper

Dash cayenne pepper
2 lb shrimp, shelled, deveined,
   and boiled for 5 minutes
   (until they just turn pink)
1/4 cup dry white wine
2 Tbsp chopped parsley

1. In a large skillet over medium heat, heat the oil. Sauté the shallots and garlic for 2 minutes.
2. Add the chopped tomato, tomato sauce, salt, pepper, and cayenne pepper. Bring to a boil, stirring occasionally.
3. Reduce the heat to low and let simmer uncovered for 10 minutes. Stir in the shrimp and wine. Continue to cook for 5 minutes.
4. Remove from the heat and transfer to a serving platter. Sprinkle with parsley and serve.

NUTRITION FACTS

8 Servings
Serving Size 2–3 oz shrimp
** with sauce**

AMOUNT PER SERVING

Exchanges
2 Lean Meat

Calories	117
Calories from Fat	38
Total Fat	4 g
Saturated Fat	1 g
Cholesterol	131 mg
Sodium	354 mg
Total Carbohydrate	4 g
Dietary Fiber	1 g
Sugars	2 g
Protein	15 g

NUTRITION FACTS

4 Servings
Serving Size 3 oz with
  topping

AMOUNT PER SERVING

Exchanges
2 Lean Meat
1 Fat

Calories	165	
Calories from Fat	94	
Total Fat	10	g
Saturated Fat	1	g
Cholesterol	41	mg
Sodium	41	mg
with added salt	331	mg
Total Carbohydrate	2	g
Dietary Fiber	1	g
Sugars	1	g
Protein	16	g

Trout Amandine

Pan-dressed trout is gutted, but with the head and tail left on.
Ask your fish market to do this for you.

2 Tbsp fresh lemon juice
1 Tbsp canola oil
2 pan-dressed trout
  (about 6–8 oz each)
1/2 tsp salt (optional)

Fresh ground pepper
2 Tbsp sliced almonds, toasted
1 lemon, cut into wedges
Parsley sprigs

1. Preheat the oven to 350 degrees. Combine the lemon juice and oil and brush the inside and outside of each fish. Sprinkle salt and pepper evenly inside each fish cavity.

2. Bake uncovered for 6 to 9 minutes or until trout is opaque and flakes easily with a fork.

3. Sprinkle with toasted almonds. Garnish with lemon wedges and parsley to serve.

Vegetable Salmon Cakes

Canned salmon is an excellent source of calcium.

1 lb canned salmon, drained

1 cup dried bread crumbs

3 medium russet or white potatoes, skinned, cooked, and mashed

1/2 cup grated carrots

1/2 cup minced onion

2 Tbsp fresh lemon juice

1/2 cup egg substitute, slightly beaten

1. In a medium bowl, combine the salmon, 1/2 cup of the bread crumbs, potatoes, carrots, onion, lemon juice, and egg substitute, mixing well.

2. Coat a large skillet with nonstick cooking spray and place over medium heat. Form the salmon into patties and coat with remaining bread crumbs.

3. Place the salmon cakes in the heated skillet and cook for 6 minutes per side or until golden brown. Remove from heat, transfer to a serving platter, and serve hot.

NUTRITION FACTS

4 Servings
Serving Size 4 oz

AMOUNT PER SERVING

Exchanges
2 1/2 Starch
2 Lean Meat

Calories	322
Calories from Fat	59
Total Fat	7 g
Saturated Fat	2 g
Cholesterol	36 mg
Sodium	729 mg
Total Carbohydrate	38 g
Dietary Fiber	3 g
Sugars	4 g
Protein	27 g

Vegetables

Artichokes Parmesan, 183

Asparagus with Vinaigrette, 184

Broccoli with Lemon Sauce, 185

Carrots Marsala, 186

Chinese Asparagus, 187

Creamed Spinach, 188

Creole Eggplant, 189

Dill-Flavored Carrots, 190

Green Beans with Garlic and Onion, 191

Herb-Broiled Tomatoes, 192

Mushroom Cassoulets, 193

Sautéed Sweet Peppers, 194

Sherried Peppers with Bean Sprouts, 195

Snow Peas with Sesame Seeds, 196

Squash and Tomato Cassoulet, 197

Tangy Green Beans, 198

Vegetable Confetti, 199

Vegetable-Stuffed Yellow Squash, 200

Zucchini and Onion Kabobs, 201

Zucchini Sauté, 202

Artichokes Parmesan

～

*These tender artichoke hearts with crumb topping
are as easy as they are elegant.*

NUTRITION FACTS
4 Servings
Serving Size 1/2 cup

AMOUNT PER SERVING

Exchanges
1/2 Starch
1 Vegetable
1/2 Fat

Calories	83
Calories from Fat	18
Total Fat	2 g
Saturated Fat	1 g
Cholesterol	2 mg
Sodium	352 mg
Total Carbohydrate	14 g
Dietary Fiber	12 g
Sugars	8 g
Protein	4 g

1/4 cup dried bread crumbs
2 Tbsp Parmesan cheese
4 Tbsp low-calorie Italian
  salad dressing (divided use)

9 oz canned and drained (packed
  in water) or frozen and thawed
  artichoke hearts
2 medium tomatoes, quartered

1. In a small bowl, combine bread crumbs, cheese, and 3 Tbsp salad dressing. Mix well and set aside.

2. In another bowl, combine artichoke hearts with remaining 1 Tbsp salad dressing, tossing thoroughly. Arrange artichoke hearts and tomato wedges in a 1-quart casserole dish.

3. Sprinkle bread crumb mixture over vegetables, and bake at 350 degrees for 35 to 40 minutes or until topping is light brown.

Asparagus with Vinaigrette

The secret to great asparagus is to cook it until it is still bright green and slightly crunchy. Look for thin asparagus with compact buds.

1 1/2 lb fresh or frozen asparagus
1/2 cup red wine vinegar
1/2 tsp dried or 1 tsp fresh tarragon
2 Tbsp fresh chives
3 Tbsp fresh chopped parsley
1/2 cup water

1 Tbsp olive oil
2 Tbsp Dijon mustard
1 lb fresh spinach leaves, trimmed
  of stems, washed, and dried
2 large tomatoes, cut into wedges

1. Place 1 inch of water in a pot, and place steamer inside. Arrange asparagus on top of steamer. Steam fresh asparagus for 4 minutes and frozen asparagus for 6 to 8 minutes. Immediately rinse asparagus under cold water to stop the cooking. (This helps keep asparagus bright green and crunchy.) Set aside.

2. In a small bowl or salad cruet, combine remaining ingredients except spinach and tomatoes. Mix or shake well.

3. Pour dressing over asparagus and refrigerate for 5 to 6 hours.

4. To serve, line plates with spinach leaves, and place asparagus on top of spinach. Garnish with tomato wedges, and spoon any remaining dressing on top.

NUTRITION FACTS
6 Servings
Serving Size 1/2 cup

AMOUNT PER SERVING

Exchanges
2 Vegetable
1/2 Fat

Calories	68	
Calories from Fat	28	
Total Fat	3	g
Saturated Fat	0	g
Cholesterol	0	mg
Sodium	127	mg
Total Carbohydrate	9	g
Dietary Fiber	4	g
Sugars	4	g
Protein	4	g

Broccoli with Lemon Sauce

Fresh broccoli only needs a little enhancement. To vary this recipe, add 1/2 tsp marjoram and 1/2 tsp dried basil to the lemon-butter mixture.

1 1/2 lb fresh broccoli florets
2 Tbsp reduced-fat margarine

2 Tbsp lemon juice
1 large lemon, cut into wedges

1. Place broccoli into a vegetable steamer basket over boiling water. Cover and simmer for 8 to 10 minutes until broccoli is just tender.

2. In a small skillet, melt margarine, then add lemon juice. Drizzle lemon butter over broccoli, and serve with lemon wedges.

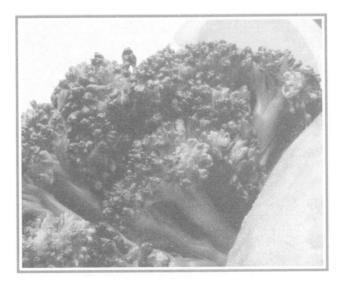

Carrots Marsala

This side dish is perfect served with an authentic Italian meal.

10 carrots (about 1 lb), peeled and
   diagonally sliced
1/4 cup Marsala wine
1/4 cup water

1 Tbsp olive oil
Fresh ground pepper
1 Tbsp fresh chopped parsley

1. In a large saucepan, combine carrots, wine, water, oil, and pepper. Bring to a boil, cover, reduce the heat, and simmer for 8 to 10 minutes until carrots are just tender, basting occasionally.
2. Transfer to a serving dish, spoon any juices on top, and sprinkle with parsley.

NUTRITION FACTS
6 Servings
Serving Size 1/2 cup

AMOUNT PER SERVING

Exchanges
1 Vegetable
1/2 Fat

Calories	53
Calories from Fat	21
Total Fat	2 g
Saturated Fat	0 g
Cholesterol	0 mg
Sodium	39 mg
Total Carbohydrate	7 g
Dietary Fiber	2 g
Sugars	3 g
Protein	1 g

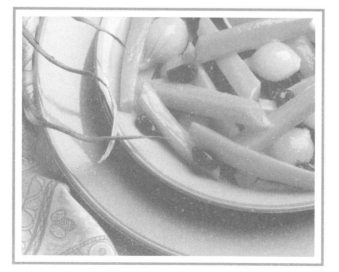

Chinese Asparagus

This is a delicious complement to any Chinese meal.

1 lb asparagus
1/2 cup low-sodium chicken broth
2 Tbsp lite soy sauce
1 Tbsp rice vinegar
2 tsp cornstarch

1 Tbsp water
1 Tbsp canola oil
2 tsp grated ginger
1 scallion, minced

1. Trim the tough ends off the asparagus. Cut stalks diagonally into 2-inch pieces.
2. In a small bowl, combine broth, soy sauce, and rice vinegar. In a measuring cup, combine cornstarch and water. Set aside.
3. Heat oil in a wok or skillet. Add ginger and scallions and stir-fry for 30 seconds. Add asparagus and stir-fry for a few seconds more. Add broth mixture and bring to a boil. Cover and simmer for 3 to 5 minutes until asparagus is just tender.
4. Add cornstarch mixture and cook until thickened. Serve.

Creamed Spinach

This may become a family favorite!

1 1/2 lb fresh spinach leaves
2 Tbsp reduced-fat margarine
2 Tbsp cornstarch
Fresh ground pepper

Dash salt
3/4 cup evaporated fat-free milk
1/4 cup egg substitute, beaten

1. Remove and discard tough spinach stems. Wash leaves thoroughly and chop. Steam the spinach for 3 to 5 minutes and set aside.
2. In a skillet, heat margarine. Blend in cornstarch, pepper, and salt. Stir constantly.
3. Add milk, bring to a boil, and stir constantly for 1 minute. Remove sauce from heat.
4. Vigorously stir about 3 Tbsp sauce into the beaten egg and immediately add this mixture back to the skillet. Add steamed spinach to the skillet and coat with sauce. Serve.

NUTRITION FACTS
4 Servings
Serving Size 1/2 cup

AMOUNT PER SERVING

Exchanges
1 Starch
1/2 Fat

Calories	105	
Calories from Fat	28	
Total Fat	3	g
Saturated Fat	1	g
Cholesterol	2	mg
Sodium	219	mg
Total Carbohydrate	13	g
Dietary Fiber	2	g
Sugars	5	g
Protein	8	g

Creole Eggplant

Instead of frying eggplant, dress it up in a tangy Creole sauce.

1 medium eggplant (about 4 oz)
2 medium garlic cloves, minced
1 large green bell pepper, chopped
1 medium onion, chopped
1/4 tsp dried thyme

1/4 tsp dried rosemary
Dash hot pepper sauce (or to taste)
1/4 tsp chili powder
10 oz no-salt-added tomato sauce

1. Peel and cube eggplant. Place in a bowl of salted water (1/2 tsp) to cover, and let eggplant stand for 1 hour. Drain and pat dry.
2. Combine all ingredients in a large skillet over low heat, mixing well. Cover and simmer for 15 to 20 minutes until vegetables are just tender. Transfer to a serving dish and serve.

Dill-Flavored Carrots

You can eat these oven-baked carrots like French fries.

10 carrots (about 1 lb), peeled
   and cut into sticks similar to
   French fries
1 Tbsp olive oil

1/4 tsp dried dill weed
Fresh ground pepper
1 Tbsp water

1. Preheat the oven to 375 degrees.
2. Place carrot sticks in the center of a large piece of aluminum foil. Add oil and sprinkle with dill weed, pepper, and water. Wrap carrots securely in foil and crimp edges.
2. Bake for 40 to 45 minutes or until carrots are just tender.

NUTRITION FACTS
6 Servings
Serving Size 1/2 cup

AMOUNT PER SERVING

Exchanges
1 Vegetable
1/2 Fat

Calories	46	
Calories from Fat	21	
Total Fat	2	g
Saturated Fat	0	g
Cholesterol	0	mg
Sodium	38	mg
Total Carbohydrate	6	g
Dietary Fiber	2	g
Sugars	2	g
Protein	1	g

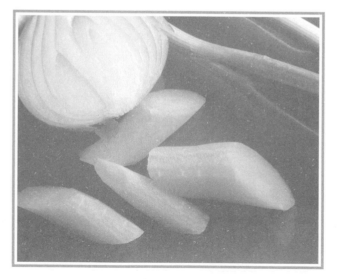

Green Beans with Garlic and Onion

This is a great side dish for Chinese food.

1 lb fresh green beans, trimmed and cut into 2-inch pieces
1 Tbsp olive oil
1 small onion, chopped

1 large garlic clove, minced
1 Tbsp white vinegar
1/4 cup Parmesan cheese
Fresh ground pepper

1. Steam beans for 7 minutes or until just tender. Set aside.

2. In a skillet, heat oil over low heat. Add onion and garlic and sauté for 4 to 5 minutes or until onion is translucent.

3. Transfer beans to a serving bowl and add onion mixture and vinegar, tossing well. Sprinkle with cheese and pepper and serve.

Herb-Broiled Tomatoes

These tomatoes are simple to fix, elegant to eat.

4 medium tomatoes

1/4 cup Parmesan cheese

2 Tbsp dried bread crumbs

2 Tbsp fresh minced parsley

1 tsp dried basil

1 tsp dried oregano

Fresh ground pepper

1 Tbsp olive oil

1. Remove stems from tomatoes and cut in half crosswise.

2. Combine remaining ingredients in a small bowl, and lightly press mixture over cut side of tomato halves.

3. Place tomatoes on a baking sheet, cut side up, and broil about 6 inches from the heat for 3 to 5 minutes or until topping is browned.

NUTRITION FACTS

8 Servings
Serving Size 1/2 tomato

AMOUNT PER SERVING

Exchanges
1 Vegetable
1/2 Fat

Calories	46	
Calories from Fat	25	
Total Fat	3	g
Saturated Fat	1	g
Cholesterol	3	mg
Sodium	38	mg
Total Carbohydrate	4	g
Dietary Fiber	1	g
Sugars	2	g
Protein	2	g

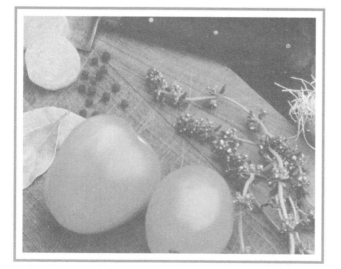

Mushroom Cassoulets

Here is a side dish that is not a bit of trouble to prepare, yet tastes delicious!

1 lb mushrooms, sliced
1 medium onion, chopped
1 cup low-sodium chicken broth
1 sprig thyme
1 sprig oregano

Leaves from 1 celery stalk
2 Tbsp lemon juice
Fresh ground pepper
1/2 cup dried bread crumbs
2 Tbsp olive oil

1. Combine mushrooms, onion, and chicken broth in a saucepan. Tie together thyme, oregano, and celery leaves and add to mushrooms.
2. Add lemon juice and pepper, and bring to a boil. Boil until liquid is reduced, about 10 minutes. Remove bundle of herbs.
3. Divide mushroom mixture equally into small ramekins. Mix bread crumbs and oil together, and sprinkle on top of each casserole.
4. Bake at 350 degrees for 20 minutes or until tops are golden brown. Remove from heat, and let cool slightly before serving.

Sautéed Sweet Peppers

Add a little chicken or shrimp, and you can turn this side dish into a main meal.

2 medium green bell peppers, cut into 1-inch squares
2 medium red bell peppers, cut into 1-inch squares
1 Tbsp olive oil

2 Tbsp water
Fresh ground pepper
1/2 tsp dried basil
2 cups precooked rice, hot

1. In a large skillet over medium heat, heat oil. Add peppers and sauté for 3 to 5 minutes, stirring frequently.

2. Add water and pepper; continue sautéing for 4 to 5 minutes or until peppers are just tender. Stir in basil and remove from heat.

3. Spread rice over a serving platter, spoon peppers and liquid on top, and serve.

NUTRITION FACTS

6 Servings
Serving Size 1/2 cup
  vegetables and about
  1/3 cup rice

AMOUNT PER SERVING

Exchanges
1 Starch
1 Vegetable

Calories	110
Calories from Fat	23
Total Fat	3 g
Saturated Fat	0 g
Cholesterol	0 mg
Sodium	3 mg
Total Carbohydrate	20 g
Dietary Fiber	2 g
Sugars	2 g
Protein	2 g

NUTRITION FACTS

4 Servings
Serving Size 1/2 cup

AMOUNT PER SERVING

Exchanges
1 Vegetable

Calories	33	
Calories from Fat	0	
Total Fat	0	g
Saturated Fat	0	g
Cholesterol	0	mg
Sodium	109	mg
Total Carbohydrate	7	g
Dietary Fiber	3	g
Sugars	1	g
Protein	2	g

Sherried Peppers with Bean Sprouts

This side dish has so many options: add carrots, snow peas, or broccoli for more vegetables, or serve over rice, noodles, or even a baked potato.

1 green bell pepper, julienned
1 red bell pepper, julienned
2 cups fresh bean sprouts

2 tsp lite soy sauce
1 Tbsp dry sherry
1 tsp red wine vinegar

1. In a large skillet over medium heat, combine peppers, bean sprouts, soy sauce, and sherry, mixing well. Cover and cook for 5 to 7 minutes or until vegetables are just tender.

2. Stir in vinegar and remove from heat. Serve hot.

Snow Peas
with Sesame Seeds

*Try these crisp snow peas with Sea Bass with Ginger Sauce
(see recipe, page 176).*

2 cups water
1 lb trimmed fresh snow peas
3 Tbsp sesame seeds

1 Tbsp chopped shallots
Fresh ground pepper

1. Boil water in a saucepan. Add snow peas and then turn off the heat. After 1 minute, rinse the snow peas under cold running water to stop the cooking process, then drain. (This method of blanching helps the snow peas to retain their bright green color and crispness.)

2. In a skillet, toast sesame seeds for 1 minute over medium heat. Add snow peas, shallots, and pepper. Continue sautéing for 1 to 2 minutes until snow peas are coated with sesame seeds. Serve.

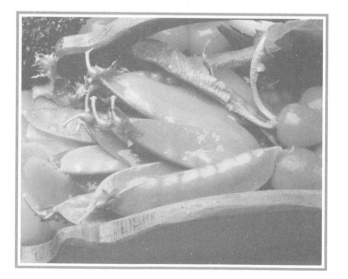

Squash and Tomato Cassoulet

Here squash and tomatoes combine in a smooth custard sauce.

1 Tbsp olive oil
6 small yellow squash, sliced
1 medium onion, minced
2 garlic cloves, minced
2 Tbsp chopped parsley

Fresh ground pepper
2 medium tomatoes, sliced
1 cup egg substitute
1 cup evaporated fat-free milk

1. Preheat the oven to 350 degrees.
2. In a large skillet over medium heat, heat oil. Add squash, onion, and garlic and sauté for 5 minutes. Add parsley and pepper.
3. Layer squash mixture and tomatoes in a casserole dish. Combine egg substitute with evaporated milk, blending well, and pour over vegetables. Bake for 20 to 25 minutes or until custard is set. Remove from oven and let cool slightly before serving.

Tangy Green Beans

Put some zing and zip into fresh green beans with this tasty side dish.

1 tsp olive oil
1 large onion, chopped
1/2 cup chopped green bell pepper
1 lb fresh green beans, trimmed

1 tsp dried tarragon
1/4 cup water
1 tsp lemon pepper

1. In a large skillet over medium heat, heat oil. Sauté onion until it is tender, about 5 or 6 minutes. Add green pepper and sauté for 5 minutes more.
2. Add green beans, tarragon, water, and lemon pepper, mixing well. Cover and simmer for 10 minutes or until beans are just tender. Transfer to a bowl and serve.

NUTRITION FACTS

6 Servings
Serving Size 1/2 cup

AMOUNT PER SERVING

Exchanges
2 Vegetable

Calories	56	
Calories from Fat	10	
Total Fat	1	g
Saturated Fat	0	g
Cholesterol	0	mg
Sodium	4	mg
Total Carbohydrate	11	g
Dietary Fiber	3	g
Sugars	3	g
Protein	2	g

Vegetable Confetti

Everything but the kitchen sink is in here, for a very nutritious side dish.

2 Tbsp olive oil
1/2 cup plus 2 Tbsp low-sodium chicken broth
1/4 cup chopped scallions
3 garlic cloves, minced
1 cup fresh broccoli, cut into florets
1 cup sliced zucchini
1 cup sliced mushrooms

1 cup cauliflower, broken into florets
3 medium potatoes, peeled and cubed
1 tsp dried oregano
1/2 tsp dried basil
1/2 tsp dried thyme
1/4 tsp paprika
Fresh ground pepper

1. Heat olive oil and 2 Tbsp of broth in a large skillet over medium heat. Add scallions and garlic and sauté for 2 minutes.

2. Add vegetables and remaining broth. Cover and simmer for 15 to 20 minutes until vegetables are just tender. Sprinkle with dried herbs and pepper and serve.

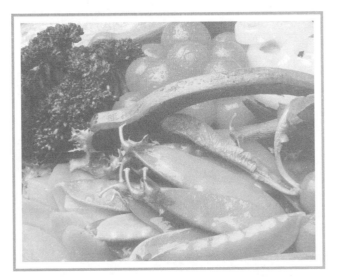

Vegetable-Stuffed Yellow Squash

Spoon rice into the squash shells, and top with yummy vegetables for a meat-free meal.

6 small yellow squash

1 tomato, finely chopped

1/2 cup minced onion

1/2 cup finely chopped green bell pepper

1/2 cup shredded low-fat cheddar cheese

Fresh ground pepper

1. Preheat the oven to 400 degrees.

2. Place squash in a large pot of boiling water. Cover, reduce heat, and simmer for 5 to 7 minutes or until squash is just tender. Drain and allow to cool slightly.

3. Trim stems from squash and cut in half lengthwise. Gently scoop out the pulp, leaving a firm shell. Drain and chop the pulp.

4. In a large mixing bowl, combine pulp and the remaining ingredients, blending well.

5. Place squash shells in a 13 × 9 × 2-inch baking dish, gently spoon vegetable mixture into shells, and bake for 15 to 20 minutes. Remove from oven and let cool slightly before serving.

NUTRITION FACTS

6 Servings
Serving Size 1 squash

AMOUNT PER SERVING

Exchanges
2 Vegetable

Calories	50	
Calories from Fat	10	
Total Fat	1	g
Saturated Fat	0	g
Cholesterol	2	mg
Sodium	62	mg
Total Carbohydrate	8	g
Dietary Fiber	2	g
Sugars	4	g
Protein	4	g

Zucchini and Onion Kabobs

Here's a nice side dish for grilled fish, chicken, or beef.

6 medium zucchini
  (about 4–5 oz each)
4 medium red onions, quartered
3/4 cup low-calorie Italian
  salad dressing

3 Tbsp lemon juice
1 large lemon, cut into wedges

1. Combine all ingredients in a large baking dish, mixing thoroughly. Cover and let marinate, refrigerated, for 2 to 3 hours.

2. Remove vegetables from marinade (reserving marinade) and alternate zucchini and onion on metal or wooden skewers (remember to soak the wooden skewers in water before using).

3. Grill kabobs 6 inches above medium heat, basting frequently, for about 20 minutes. Transfer to a platter, and garnish with lemon wedges. Serve with remaining marinade.

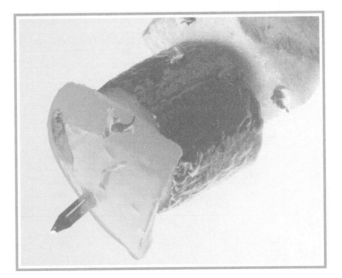

Zucchini Sauté

~

Red onion gives this zucchini a sweetness that is irresistible.

1 Tbsp olive oil
1 medium red onion, chopped
3 medium zucchini (about 5–6 oz each), cut into rounds

1/4 tsp dried oregano
Fresh ground pepper

1. In a large skillet over medium heat, heat oil. Add onion and sauté until onion is translucent but not browned.
2. Add zucchini, cover, and simmer 3 to 4 minutes. Sprinkle with oregano and pepper, and serve hot.

NUTRITION FACTS

4 Servings
Serving Size 1/2 cup

AMOUNT PER SERVING

Exchanges
1 Vegetable
1 Fat

Calories	62	
Calories from Fat	31	
Total Fat	3	g
Saturated Fat	0	g
Cholesterol	0	mg
Sodium	4	mg
Total Carbohydrate	8	g
Dietary Fiber	2	g
Sugars	5	g
Protein	1	g

Rice & Potatoes

Asian Fried Rice, 205

Baked Potato Toppers, 206

Colorful Rice Casserole, 207

Curried Rice with Pineapple, 208

Festive Sweet Potatoes, 209

Potato Parmesan Chips, 210

Rice Parmesan, 211

Rice with Spinach and Feta, 212

Sage Potatoes, 213

Scalloped Potatoes, 214

Asian Fried Rice

Now you can make this traditional favorite at home!

2 Tbsp peanut oil
1/4 cup chopped onion
1/2 cup sliced carrot
2 Tbsp chopped green bell pepper
2 cups cooked rice, cold
1/2 cup water chestnuts, drained
1/2 cup sliced mushrooms
2 Tbsp lite soy sauce
3/4 cup egg substitute, beaten
1/2 cup sliced scallions

1. In a large skillet, heat oil. Sauté onion, carrot, and green pepper for 5 to 6 minutes.
2. Stir in rice, water chestnuts, mushrooms, and soy sauce, and stir-fry for 8 to 10 minutes.
3. Stir in egg substitute and continue to stir-fry for another 3 minutes. Top with sliced scallions to serve.

Baked Potato Toppers

Try these ideas to spice up your spud! Start by baking an 8-ounce potato for about 50 to 60 minutes in a 350-degree oven.

Create a pizza potato: add 2 Tbsp of your favorite tomato sauce and 1 Tbsp Parmesan cheese. Place potato in oven to melt cheese.

NUTRITION FACTS			
AMOUNT PER SERVING			
	Calories	233	
	Calories from Fat	16	
Exchanges	Total Fat	2g	
3 Starch	Saturated Fat	1g	
	Cholesterol	4mg	
	Sodium	285mg	
	Total Carbohydrate	49g	
	Dietary Fiber	5g	
	Sugars	4g	
	Protein	7g	

Spruce it up with herbs: add 1 Tbsp low-fat sour cream and 1 tsp chopped chives, thyme, rosemary, or scallions.

NUTRITION FACTS

AMOUNT PER SERVING

Exchanges
3 Starch

Calories 222
Calories from Fat 11
Total Fat 1g
Saturated Fat 1g
Cholesterol 0mg
Sodium 35mg

Total Carbohydrate 48g
Dietary Fiber 4g
Sugars 5g
Protein 5g

For a main meal: add 1/4 cup chopped cooked chicken mixed with 2 Tbsp salsa.

NUTRITION FACTS

AMOUNT PER SERVING

Exchanges
3 Starch
1 Lean Meat

Calories 278
Calories from Fat 16
Total Fat 2g
Saturated Fat 0g
Cholesterol 36mg
Sodium 127mg

Total Carbohydrate 48g
Dietary Fiber 5g
Sugars 4g
Protein 18g

Colorful Rice Casserole

Enjoy this recipe when zucchini are at their freshest.

1 Tbsp olive oil
1 1/2 lb zucchini, thinly sliced
3/4 cup chopped scallions
2 cups corn kernels (frozen or fresh; if frozen, defrost)
1 16-oz can no-salt-added chopped tomatoes, undrained
1/4 cup chopped parsley
1 tsp oregano
3 cups cooked rice (white or brown)

1. In a large skillet, heat oil. Add zucchini and scallions and sauté for 5 minutes.

2. Add remaining ingredients, cover, reduce heat, and simmer for 10 to 15 minutes or until vegetables are heated through. Transfer to a bowl and serve.

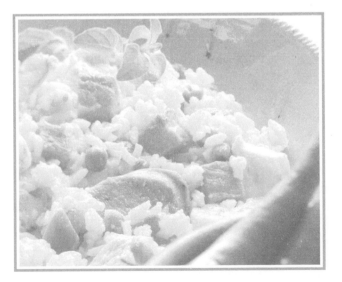

Curried Rice with Pineapple

Sweet pineapple sparks the flavor in this side dish.

1 onion, chopped
1 1/2 cups water
1 1/4 cups low-sodium beef broth
1 cup uncooked rice

1 tsp curry powder
1/4 tsp garlic powder
8 oz pineapple chunks, drained

1. In a medium saucepan, combine onion, water, and beef broth. Bring to a boil, and add rice, curry powder, and garlic powder. Cover and reduce heat. Simmer for 25 minutes.

2. Add pineapple and continue to simmer 5 to 7 minutes more until rice is tender and water is absorbed. Transfer to a serving bowl and serve.

NUTRITION FACTS

4 Servings
Serving Size about 1/2 cup

AMOUNT PER SERVING

Exchanges
3 Starch

Calories	215
Calories from Fat	8
Total Fat	1 g
Saturated Fat	0 g
Cholesterol	0 mg
Sodium	21 mg
Total Carbohydrate	46 g
Dietary Fiber	2 g
Sugars	7 g
Protein	5 g

Festive Sweet Potatoes

~

Forget gobs of brown sugar and butter.
Pineapple and spices add flavor, not fat.

4 sweet potatoes (about 20 oz total)
2 cups crushed pineapple in
   its own juice

2 tsp cinnamon
1 tsp nutmeg
1 Tbsp slivered almonds

1. In a large saucepan, boil potatoes over medium heat for about 45 minutes until you can pierce them easily with a fork (or bake them directly on a rack in a preheated 350-degree oven for 45 minutes).

2. Let potatoes cool, then gently peel them. Mash potatoes with pineapple and spices and place in a casserole dish coated with nonstick cooking spray.

3. Top casserole with almonds and bake for 20 minutes at 350 degrees.

Potato Parmesan Chips

These tasty and colorful chips are a change from the usual plain potato chips.

4 large potatoes (4–5 oz each)
2 Tbsp olive oil
1 tsp grated onion
Dash salt

Fresh ground pepper
1/4 tsp paprika
2 Tbsp Parmesan cheese

1. Wash and cut unpeeled potatoes into 1/8-inch-thick slices. Place in a single layer over baking sheets coated with cooking spray.
2. Heat oil in a small skillet and add onion, salt, pepper, and paprika. Brush potatoes with oil mixture and bake at 425 degrees for 15 to 20 minutes or until potatoes are crispy and golden brown.
3. Remove from oven and sprinkle with cheese. Serve.

NUTRITION FACTS

8 Servings
Serving Size 1/2 potato

AMOUNT PER SERVING

Exchanges
1 Starch
1/2 Fat

Calories	105	
Calories from Fat	34	
Total Fat	4	g
Saturated Fat	1	g
Cholesterol	1	mg
Sodium	46	mg
Total Carbohydrate	16	g
Dietary Fiber	2	g
Sugars	1	g
Protein	2	g

Rice Parmesan

You can probably make this dish anytime with ingredients you have on hand.

1 Tbsp canola oil
1 medium onion, chopped
1 garlic clove, minced
1 cup low-sodium chicken broth

1 cup uncooked rice
1/2 cup dry white wine
1/3 cup grated fresh Parmesan
  cheese

1. In a skillet over medium heat, heat oil. Add onion and garlic and sauté for 8 minutes.
2. Stir in chicken broth, rice, and wine and bring to a boil. Reduce heat to low, cover, and continue cooking for 20 to 25 minutes or until liquid is absorbed.
3. Transfer to a serving bowl and sprinkle with cheese before serving.

Rice with Spinach and Feta

Here's rice with a Greek twist.

1 cup uncooked rice

1 cup low-sodium chicken broth

1 cup water

1 Tbsp olive oil

1 medium onion, chopped

1 cup sliced mushrooms

2 garlic cloves, minced

1 Tbsp lemon juice

1/2 tsp dried oregano

6 cups fresh spinach, stems trimmed, washed, patted dry, and coarsely chopped

1/2 cup crumbled fat-free feta cheese

Fresh ground pepper

1. In a medium saucepan over medium heat, combine rice, chicken broth, and water. Bring to a boil, cover, reduce heat, and simmer for 15 minutes. Transfer to a serving bowl.

2. In a skillet, heat oil. Sauté onion, mushrooms, and garlic for 5 to 7 minutes. Stir in lemon juice and oregano. Add spinach, cheese, and pepper, tossing until spinach is slightly wilted.

3. Toss with rice and serve.

NUTRITION FACTS

5 Servings
Serving Size 1/2 cup

AMOUNT PER SERVING

Exchanges
2 Starch
1 Vegetable
1/2 Fat

Calories	216	
Calories from Fat	32	
Total Fat	4	g
Saturated Fat	1	g
Cholesterol	1	mg
Sodium	417	mg
Total Carbohydrate	37	g
Dietary Fiber	2	g
Sugars	3	g
Protein	10	g

Exchanges
1 Starch
1 1/2 Fat

Calories	142
Calories from Fat	62
Total Fat	7 g
Saturated Fat	1 g
Cholesterol	0 mg
Sodium	6 mg
Total Carbohydrate	19 g
Dietary Fiber	2 g
Sugars	3 g
Protein	2 g

Sage Potatoes

This dish is a good addition to your brunch table.

2 Tbsp olive oil
1 small onion, chopped
1 garlic clove, minced
1 tsp dried sage

2 potatoes (4–5 oz each), unpeeled,
halved lengthwise, and sliced
crosswise into thin slices

1. In a large skillet over medium heat, heat oil. Add onion and garlic and sauté for 2 to 3 minutes.
2. Add sage and potatoes, cover, and cook for 10 minutes, stirring occasionally.
3. Turn potatoes over with a spatula, and continue to cook for another 5 to 7 minutes until golden brown. Serve.

Scalloped Potatoes

These potatoes are still creamy and rich, but with far less fat.

6 small potatoes (4 oz each),
   unpeeled
4 cups water
1 tsp olive oil
1/3 cup chopped onion
1/2 cup egg substitute

1 cup fat-free sour cream
1/4 tsp salt
Fresh ground pepper
1/2 cup shredded reduced-fat mild
   cheddar cheese

1. Wash potatoes and place in a saucepan with water. Bring to a boil, lower the heat, and let potatoes cook for 25 minutes. Drain potatoes, let cool, and slice into 1/4-inch slices.
2. Heat oil in a skillet. Add onion and sauté for 5 minutes. Add onion to egg substitute, sour cream, salt, and pepper in a bowl and mix well.
3. Lay potato slices in a casserole dish. Spoon sour cream mixture over potatoes. Top with cheese.
4. Bake for 35 minutes at 350 degrees until top is browned.

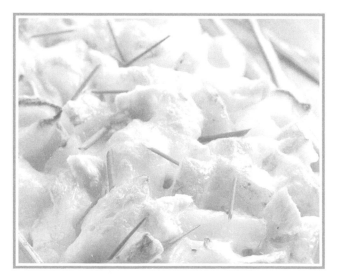

AMOUNT PER SERVING

Exchanges
1 Starch
1 Lean Meat

Calories	130
Calories from Fat	19
Total Fat	2 g
Saturated Fat	1 g
Cholesterol	8 mg
Sodium	179 mg
Total Carbohydrate	18 g
Dietary Fiber	2 g
Sugars	3 g
Protein	7 g

Breads & Muffins

Banana Carrot Muffins, 217

Blueberry Scones, 218

Buttermilk Biscuits, 219

Corn Muffins, 220

Cranberry-Orange Scones, 221

Date Nut Bread, 222

Homemade Seasoned Bread Crumbs, 223

Irish Soda Bread, 224

Pineapple Muffins, 225

Spoon Bread, 226

Sweet Potato and Zucchini Bread, 227

Banana Carrot Muffins

These muffins are moist, sweet, and full of good-for-you ingredients!

1 1/2 cups whole-wheat or
  unbleached flour
2 tsp baking powder
1 tsp baking soda
1/2 tsp nutmeg
Pinch cloves
1/2 cup egg substitute

1/2 cup unsweetened applesauce
2 Tbsp fructose
1/2 cup low-fat buttermilk
1/2 cup mashed banana
1 cup grated carrot
1 tsp vanilla

1. Preheat the oven to 400 degrees. Combine the flour, baking powder, baking soda, nutmeg, and cloves in a large bowl.

2. Combine the remaining ingredients in a smaller bowl. Combine all ingredients together and mix well, but do not overbeat.

3. Spoon into muffin cups and bake for 20 minutes. Serve warm or at room temperature.

NUTRITION FACTS

12 Servings
Serving Size 1 muffin

AMOUNT PER SERVING

Exchanges
1 Starch

Calories	88
Calories from Fat	3
Total Fat	0 g
Saturated Fat	0 g
Cholesterol	0 mg
Sodium	149 mg
Total Carbohydrate	18 g
Dietary Fiber	1 g
Sugars	5 g
Protein	3 g

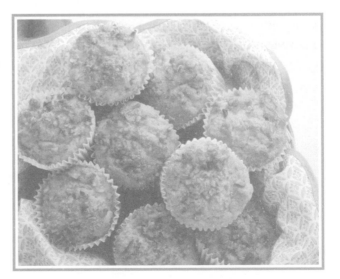

Blueberry Scones

Typical store-bought scones have a lot more fat and calories than these.

1/2 cup buttermilk at room
    temperature
3/4 cup orange juice
Grated peel of 1 orange
2 1/4 cups whole-wheat pastry flour
    or unbleached white flour

1 tsp baking soda
1 tsp cream of tartar
3 Tbsp fructose
2 Tbsp reduced-fat margarine, cold
1 cup fresh or frozen (thawed)
    blueberries

1. Preheat the oven to 375 degrees. In a small bowl, combine buttermilk, orange juice, and orange peel. Set aside.

2. Sift together flour, baking soda, cream of tartar, and fructose into a large bowl. Using a fork or pastry blender, cut in the margarine until well combined.

3. Stir in buttermilk mixture and blueberries, and mix gently by hand until well combined.

4. Turn batter onto a lightly floured cookie sheet and pat into a circle about 3/4 inch thick and 8 inches across. Using a sharp knife, cut the circle into 8 wedges, cutting almost all the way through.

5. Bake for 25 minutes until lightly browned. Cool and cut completely through the wedges to serve.

NUTRITION FACTS
8 Servings
Serving Size 1 scone

AMOUNT PER SERVING

Exchanges
2 Starch

Calories	168	
Calories from Fat	20	
Total Fat	2	g
Saturated Fat	0	g
Cholesterol	1	mg
Sodium	144	mg
Total Carbohydrate	33	g
Dietary Fiber	5	g
Sugars	9	g
Protein	5	g

Buttermilk Biscuits

These biscuits are great with thick, chunky stews.

2 cups whole-wheat pastry flour or
   unbleached white flour
1 Tbsp baking powder

1/2 tsp baking soda
1 cup low-fat buttermilk
3 Tbsp canola oil

1. Preheat the oven to 425 degrees. Lightly spray two cookie sheets with nonstick cooking spray.

2. In a medium bowl, combine the flour, baking powder, and baking soda. Add the buttermilk and oil; mix with a fork until well blended.

3. Drop the dough by heaping tablespoonfuls onto cookie sheets, 1 1/2 inches apart. Bake for 10 to 12 minutes until lightly browned.

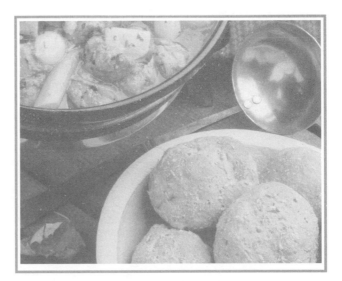

Corn Muffins

Use some of the variations included below to create interesting corn muffins. (The variations do not significantly alter the nutrient exchange information.)

1 cup yellow cornmeal
1/2 tsp baking soda
1/2 tsp baking powder
1/4 tsp salt (optional)

1 cup low-fat buttermilk
1/4 cup egg substitute
1 Tbsp canola oil

1. Preheat the oven to 425 degrees. Combine the cornmeal, baking soda, baking powder, and salt; mix thoroughly. Stir in buttermilk, egg substitute, and oil; blend well.

2. Coat muffin pans with nonstick cooking spray. Spoon batter into muffin pans, filling the cups 2/3 full. Bake for 10 to 12 minutes or until tops are golden brown. Serve warm.

Variations: add 1/2 cup cooked corn kernels, 1/2 cup finely diced green or red bell pepper, or 1/2 cup finely diced sautéd onions to the batter.

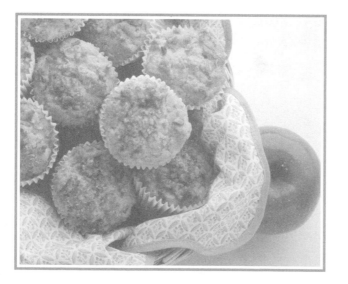

Exchanges
1 Starch

Calories	164
Calories from Fat	14
Total Fat	2 g
Saturated Fat	0 g
Cholesterol	1 mg
Sodium	76 mg
with added salt	120 mg
Total Carbohydrate	10 g
Dietary Fiber	1 g
Sugars	1 g
Protein	2 g

Cranberry-Orange Scones

These scones—low in fat and homemade—are wonderful with soup or salad.

1/2 cup dried cranberries

2 Tbsp fructose

1/2 cup low-fat buttermilk, room temperature

3/4 cup fresh orange juice

Grated peel of 1 large orange

2 1/4 cups whole-wheat pastry flour or unbleached flour

1 tsp baking soda

1 tsp cream of tartar

1/2 tsp salt

2 Tbsp reduced-fat margarine, cold

1. Preheat the oven to 375 degrees. Sprinkle a cookie sheet with flour. Soak the dried cranberries in boiling water for 5 minutes. Drain and set aside.

2. In a small bowl, mix together the fructose and buttermilk. Add orange juice and rind.

3. Sift flour, baking soda, cream of tartar, and salt in a large bowl. Using a fork or your fingers, cut in the margarine until well combined.

4. Stir the buttermilk mixture and cranberries into flour mixture and mix very gently by hand until combined.

5. Turn out the batter onto the floured cookie sheet and pat into a circle about 3/4 inch thick, 8 inches across. Using a sharp knife, cut the circle into 8 wedges, cutting almost all the way through.

6. Place the pan in the oven and bake for 25 minutes. Cool and cut completely through the wedges to serve.

Date Nut Bread

This bread tastes great with fruit or chicken salads.

1 3/4 cups chopped, pitted dates
1 1/4 cups boiling water
2 1/4 cups whole-wheat flour
1/2 cup chopped walnuts
1 tsp baking soda

1/4 cup egg substitute
1/2 cup unsweetened applesauce
2 Tbsp fructose
1 tsp vanilla or almond extract

1. In a bowl, combine the dates and boiling water; let stand for 15 minutes.

2. Preheat the oven to 350 degrees. Lightly coat a 9 × 5-inch loaf pan with nonstick cooking spray.

3. In a large bowl, combine the flour, nuts, and baking soda. Add the egg substitute, applesauce, fructose, and extract. Add the dates and mix well.

4. Pour mixture into the prepared pan and bake for 65 minutes or until a toothpick inserted in the center comes out clean.

5. Cool in the pan on a rack for 10 minutes. Remove from the pan and serve warm or cold.

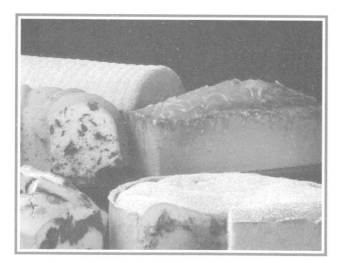

NUTRITION FACTS

16 Servings
Serving Size 1 slice

AMOUNT PER SERVING

Exchanges
1 Starch
1 Fruit

Calories	140
Calories from Fat	23
Total Fat	3 g
Saturated Fat	0 g
Cholesterol	0 mg
Sodium	58 mg
Total Carbohydrate	28 g
Dietary Fiber	4 g
Sugars	14 g
Protein	3 g

NUTRITION FACTS

8 Servings
Serving Size 1/4 cup

AMOUNT PER SERVING

Exchanges
1/2 Starch

Calories	43
Calories from Fat	5
Total Fat	1 g
Saturated Fat	0 g
Cholesterol	0 mg
Sodium	158 mg
Total Carbohydrate	9 g
Dietary Fiber	2 g
Sugars	1 g
Protein	2 g

Homemade Seasoned Bread Crumbs

These homemade seasoned bread crumbs are much lower in sodium than the store-bought variety, and are very easy to make! You can use them in any recipe calling for bread crumbs to further lower the recipe's sodium count.

1/3 16-oz loaf reduced-calorie white bread
2 tsp garlic powder
1 tsp dried basil
1 tsp dried oregano

1 tsp onion powder
1/4 tsp paprika
1/4 tsp salt
1/4 tsp pepper

1. Leave the bread out on the kitchen counter to dry for 2 days.
2. Tear the bread into bite-sized pieces and place it in a food processor or blender. Add spices and process to make crumbs.

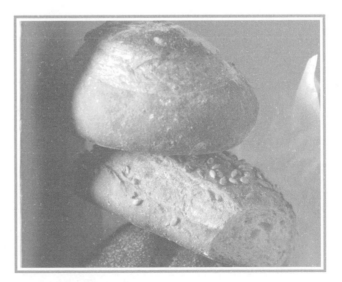

Irish Soda Bread

There is nothing like warm Irish soda bread!

2 cups unbleached white flour
1 tsp baking soda
2 Tbsp reduced-fat margarine,
chilled and cut into bits

1 Tbsp caraway seeds
1/4 cup dried currants or raisins
1 cup low-fat buttermilk

1. Preheat the oven to 375 degrees. Combine the flour and baking soda. With 2 knives or a pastry blender, work in the margarine until the mixture resembles coarse crumbs.

2. Toss in the caraway seeds and currants. With a fork, mix in the buttermilk and mix until just blended. Turn the dough out onto a lightly floured surface and knead very gently for 20 strokes, just until smooth. Do not overwork the dough.

3. Pat well into a 9-inch pan or shape well on a baking sheet. Make a shallow 4-inch cross in the center of the loaf and bake for 25 to 30 minutes until golden. Serve warm.

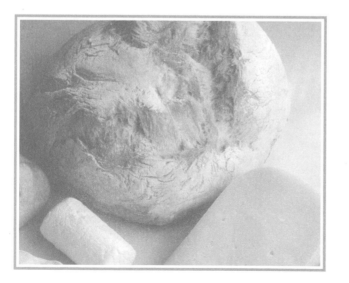

NUTRITION FACTS
10 Servings
Serving Size 1 slice

AMOUNT PER SERVING

Exchanges
1 1/2 Starch

Calories	122
Calories from Fat	14
Total Fat	2 g
Saturated Fat	0 g
Cholesterol	1 mg
Sodium	127 mg
Total Carbohydrate	23 g
Dietary Fiber	1 g
Sugars	4 g
Protein	4 g

Pineapple Muffins

These are a welcome addition to the breakfast table.
Just add fruit or juice and yogurt.

1 1/2 cups whole-wheat or pastry
  flour
2 tsp baking powder
1/2 tsp baking soda
1/4 cup fructose
2 tsp cinnamon

1/2 cup egg substitute
2/3 cup unsweetened applesauce
1 cup crushed canned pineapple,
  drained
1/2 cup diced dried apricots

1. In a medium bowl, combine dry ingredients.

2. In a large bowl, combine remaining ingredients. Slowly add dry ingredients to wet ingredients and mix until blended. Do not beat.

3. Place batter into prepared muffin cups, filling 2/3 full.

4. Bake at 350 degrees for 25 minutes until golden brown.

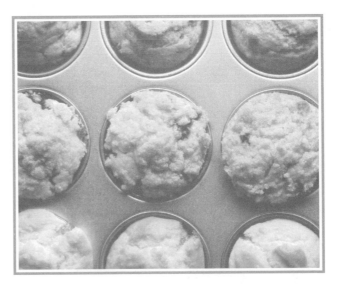

Spoon Bread

Old-fashioned spoon bread is great with any meal!

2 cups water (divided use)
2 cups yellow cornmeal
2 tsp baking powder
1 tsp salt (optional)

1 1/2 tsp baking soda
2 cups fat-free milk
1/2 cup egg substitute

1. In a bowl, combine 1 cup water with the cornmeal, baking powder, salt, and baking soda.

2. In a 3-quart saucepan, heat the remaining 1 cup water to boiling; reduce the heat to low and stir in the cornmeal mixture. Cook the mixture until thick and remove from heat.

3. Preheat the oven to 350 degrees. Lightly spray a 2-quart casserole dish with nonstick cooking spray. First add the milk, then the egg substitute, to the cornmeal mixture and beat until smooth. Pour into the casserole dish. Bake for 1 hour until set; serve warm.

NUTRITION FACTS
16 Servings
Serving Size 1/2 cup

AMOUNT PER SERVING

Exchanges
1 Starch

Calories	79	
Calories from Fat	3	
Total Fat	0	g
Saturated Fat	0	g
Cholesterol	1	mg
Sodium	142	mg
with added salt	276	mg
Total Carbohydrate	15	g
Dietary Fiber	1	g
Sugars	1	g
Protein	3	g

Sweet Potato and Zucchini Bread

This fiber-rich, slightly spicy bread is especially good around holiday time.

2 cups whole-wheat or unbleached flour
1 tsp baking powder
1/2 tsp baking soda
2 tsp cinnamon
3/4 cup egg substitute
3/4 cup unsweetened applesauce
1/4 cup fructose
1 tsp vanilla extract
1 1/2 cups grated zucchini, unpeeled
1 1/2 cups grated raw sweet potato, peeled

1. Preheat the oven to 350 degrees. Spray a 9 × 5 × 3-inch loaf pan with nonstick cooking spray and set aside.

2. Combine the flour, baking powder, baking soda, and cinnamon in a medium bowl. In a larger bowl, beat together the egg substitute, applesauce, fructose, and vanilla. Mix in the zucchini and sweet potatoes. Add the flour mixture to the bowl and mix well.

3. Transfer the batter to the prepared pan; bake for 1 hour and 15 minutes. Cool bread in the pan for 15 minutes. Turn bread onto a rack and cool completely. Slice and serve.

Breakfasts

Baked French Toast with Raspberry Sauce, 231

Fresh Blueberry Pancakes, 232

Fruit Puff Pancake, 233

Griddle Corn Cakes, 234

Hash Browns, 235

Italian Frittata, 236

Mini Breakfast Quiches, 237

Turkey Sausage Patties, 238

Western Omelet, 239

NUTRITION FACTS

4 Servings
Serving Size 2 slices

AMOUNT PER SERVING

Exchanges
2 1/2 Starch

Calories	216
Calories from Fat	25
Total Fat	3 g
Saturated Fat	1 g
Cholesterol	1 mg
Sodium	400 mg
Total Carbohydrate	38 g
Dietary Fiber	8 g
Sugars	8 g
Protein	12 g

Baked French Toast with Raspberry Sauce

This is a great version of French toast that you soak overnight in a tasty batter and let puff up in the oven.

1 cup egg substitute

2/3 cup fat-free milk

1 tsp maple extract

1 tsp cinnamon

1/2 tsp nutmeg

8 slices whole-wheat bread

2 cups frozen or fresh raspberries

1 Tbsp orange juice

1 tsp vanilla extract

2 tsp cornstarch

1. Beat together egg substitute, milk, maple extract, cinnamon, and nutmeg in a medium bowl.

2. In a casserole dish, lay bread slices side by side. Pour on the egg-milk mixture, cover, and place in refrigerator overnight.

3. The next day, bake the French toast at 350 degrees for about 30 minutes until golden brown and slightly puffed.

4. To make raspberry sauce, puree raspberries in a blender. Strain to remove seeds.

5. In a small saucepan, combine pureed berries with orange juice, vanilla, and cornstarch. Bring to a boil and cook for 1 minute until mixture is thickened. Serve over French toast.

Fresh Blueberry Pancakes

What's breakfast without a stack of warm blueberry pancakes?

1 cup flour
1/2 tsp baking soda
1 1/2 tsp baking powder
1/4 cup egg substitute

1 cup low-fat buttermilk
1 Tbsp canola oil
1/2 cup fresh blueberries,
  washed and drained

1. Combine dry ingredients in a medium-sized bowl and set aside.

2. In a small bowl, combine egg substitute, buttermilk, and oil and mix well. Add mixture to the dry ingredients, stirring until moistened, then gently fold in the blueberries.

3. Coat a griddle or skillet with cooking spray. Pour 2 Tbsp of batter for each pancake onto a hot griddle. Turn the pancakes when tops are covered with tiny bubbles and edges are golden brown.

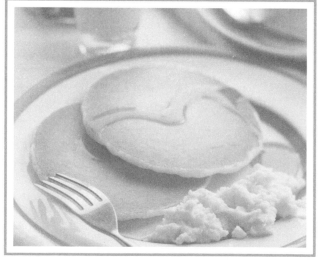

NUTRITION FACTS

8 Servings
Serving Size 2 4-inch
  pancakes

AMOUNT PER SERVING

Exchanges
1 Starch
1/2 Fat

Calories	94
Calories from Fat	20
Total Fat	2 g
Saturated Fat	0 g
Cholesterol	1 mg
Sodium	153 mg
Total Carbohydrate	15 g
Dietary Fiber	1 g
Sugars	3 g
Protein	3 g

Fruit Puff Pancake

This recipe is elegant to serve at brunch.

1 1/4 cups egg substitute
1/2 cup fat-free milk
1/2 cup flour
1 Tbsp vanilla extract

4 cups mixed fresh fruit
(try sliced strawberries,
blueberries, and bananas)

1. Preheat the oven to 425 degrees. Spray a pie plate or oven-proof skillet with nonstick cooking spray.

2. In a large bowl, combine the egg substitute and milk. Add the flour and vanilla.

3. Pour the batter into the prepared pan and place it in the oven. Bake for 15 to 20 minutes until batter is puffed and edges are browned.

4. Remove the puff pancake, fill the center with the fruit, cut into wedges, and serve.

Griddle Corn Cakes

These are not only good for breakfast, but for a light dinner with some lean ham.

2/3 cup unbleached white flour
1/3 cup whole-wheat or pastry flour
2 tsp baking powder
1 Tbsp fructose
3/4 cup buttermilk

1/4 cup egg substitute
2 Tbsp canola oil
1 cup corn kernels (frozen or fresh; if frozen, defrost)

1. Combine all dry ingredients in a medium bowl.

2. In another bowl, combine buttermilk, egg substitute, and oil. Stir in corn kernels. Slowly add this mixture to dry ingredients, just to blend. A few lumps will remain.

3. On a heated nonstick griddle, pour 1/4 cup batter per cake. Cook cakes for about 3 minutes, flip them over, and cook 1 to 2 minutes more, until golden brown. Serve.

NUTRITION FACTS
6 Servings
Serving Size 2 4-inch cakes

AMOUNT PER SERVING

Exchanges
1 1/2 Starch
1 Fat

Calories	161
Calories from Fat	47
Total Fat	5 g
Saturated Fat	1 g
Cholesterol	1 mg
Sodium	151 mg
Total Carbohydrate	24 g
Dietary Fiber	2 g
Sugars	4 g
Protein	5 g

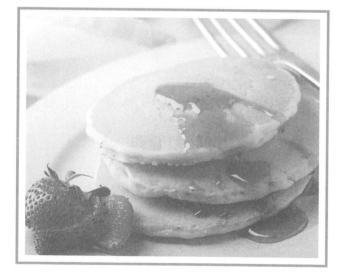

Hash Browns

~

Love hash browns, but not the fat content?
Don't worry with these greaseless, yet tasty, potatoes.

2 large baking potatoes
   (about 10 oz each)
2 Tbsp minced onion

1 tsp garlic powder
1/2 tsp dried thyme
Fresh ground pepper

1. Peel and shred each potato with a hand grater or a food processor with grater attachment. Combine potatoes with onion and spices.

2. Coat a large skillet with cooking spray and place over medium heat until hot.

3. Pack potato mixture firmly into skillet; cook mixture for 6 to 8 minutes or until bottom is browned. Invert potato patty onto a plate and return to the skillet, cooked side up.

4. Continue cooking over medium heat for another 6 to 8 minutes until bottom is browned. Remove from heat and cut into 4 wedges.

Italian Frittata

You can serve this open-faced egg dish for a casual Sunday brunch.

1/2 tsp olive oil
1 1/4 cups egg substitute
2 cups mixed steamed vegetables
(try chopped broccoli, asparagus,
and red bell peppers)
2 tsp minced garlic

2 Tbsp minced chives
1 tsp dried oregano
1 tsp dried basil
Fresh ground pepper
1/4 cup fresh grated Parmesan
cheese

1. Preheat the oven to 350 degrees. Add the oil to an ovenproof skillet or
   pie plate. In a large bowl, combine the remaining ingredients and add to
   the skillet.

2. Set the skillet in the oven and bake the frittata for 14 to 17 minutes until
   set. Remove from the oven and loosen edges with a spatula. Sprinkle
   with grated cheese, cut into wedges, and serve.

NUTRITION FACTS
4 Servings
Serving Size 1/4 recipe

AMOUNT PER SERVING

Exchanges
1 Vegetable
1 Lean Meat

Calories	82	
Calories from Fat	20	
Total Fat	2	g
Saturated Fat	1	g
Cholesterol	4	mg
Sodium	203	mg
Total Carbohydrate	6	g
Dietary Fiber	3	g
Sugars	3	g
Protein	10	g

Mini Breakfast Quiches

You can also serve these mini quiches as an appetizer.

4 oz diced green chilies
1/4 cup diced pimiento
3 cups precooked white rice
1/2 cup egg substitute
1/3 cup fat-free milk

1/2 tsp cumin
Dash salt and pepper
1 cup shredded low-fat cheddar
cheese (divided use)

1. Preheat the oven to 400 degrees. In a large mixing bowl, combine all ingredients except 1/2 cup of the cheese.

2. Spoon mixture evenly into muffin cups and sprinkle with remaining cheese. Bake for 12 to 15 minutes or until set. Carefully remove the quiches from the pan, arrange on a platter, and serve.

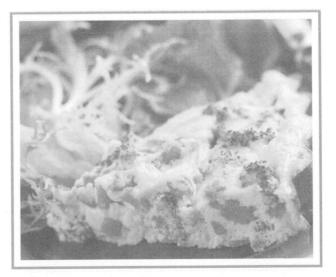

Turkey Sausage Patties

Prepare these one day in advance, and the flavor will be even better.

1/2 lb extra-lean ground turkey breast
2 Tbsp low-sodium beef broth
1/2 Tbsp lemon juice
2 Tbsp dried bread crumbs
1/8 tsp fennel seeds

1/8 tsp ground ginger
1/2 tsp grated lemon peel
1/4 tsp fresh minced sage
Fresh ground pepper
1/8 tsp ground red pepper

1. In a large bowl, combine all ingredients except cooking spray; cover and set aside for at least 15 to 20 minutes (refrigerate if overnight).
2. Coat a large skillet with cooking spray and place over medium heat until hot.
3. Shape mixture into 4 patties and place in hot skillet. Fry patties for 5 to 6 minutes on each side, remove, and let drain on paper towels.
4. Transfer to serving platter and serve while hot.

NUTRITION FACTS

4 Servings
Serving Size 2 oz

AMOUNT PER SERVING

Exchanges
2 Very Lean Meat

Calories	75	
Calories from Fat	5	
Total Fat	1	g
Saturated Fat	0	g
Cholesterol	37	mg
Sodium	52	mg
Total Carbohydrate	3	g
Dietary Fiber	0	g
Sugars	0	g
Protein	14	g

Western Omelet

*Here's a good basic omelet recipe—
experiment with your favorite vegetables.*

NUTRITION FACTS

2 Servings
Serving Size 1/2 omelet

AMOUNT PER SERVING

Exchanges
2 Lean Meat

Calories	96	
Calories from Fat	39	
Total Fat	4	g
Saturated Fat	1	g
Cholesterol	8	mg
Sodium	379	mg
Total Carbohydrate	3	g
Dietary Fiber	0	g
Sugars	2	g
Protein	11	g

1 1/2 tsp canola oil

3/4 cup egg substitute

1/4 cup minced lean ham

2 Tbsp minced green bell pepper

2 Tbsp minced onion

Dash salt

Fresh ground pepper

1. In a medium nonstick skillet over medium-low heat, heat the oil.

2. In a small mixing bowl, beat egg substitute slightly and add remaining ingredients. Pour egg mixture into heated skillet.

3. When omelet begins to set, gently lift the edges of omelet with a spatula and tilt skillet to allow uncooked portion to flow underneath. Continue cooking until eggs are firm, then transfer to serving platter.

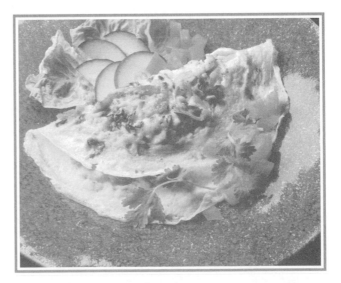

Desserts

Apple Bread Pudding, 243

Apple Cranberry Crisp, 244

Banana Pineapple Freeze, 245

Bananas Foster, 246

Basic Crêpes, 247

Basic Crêpes with Fruit Filling, 248

Carrot Cake, 249

Cherry Cheesecake, 250

Cherry Cobbler, 251

Cherry Pie, 252

Cherry Soufflé, 253

Chocolate Chip Cookies, 254

Chocolate Cupcakes, 255

Chocolate Rum Pie, 256

Cream Cheese Cookies, 257

Crêpes Suzette, 258

Crumb Pie Shell, 259

Fresh Apple Pie, 260

Graham Kerr's Basic Pie Crust, 261

Low-Calorie, Fat-Free Whipped Cream, 262

Low-Fat Cream Cheese Frosting, 263

Oatmeal Raisin Cookies, 264

Peach Crumb Cobbler, 265

Peach Shortcake, 266

Peanut Butter Cookies, 267

Pineapple Pear Medley, 268

Pumpkin Mousse, 269

Sponge Cake, 270

Strawberries Romanoff, 271

Strawberries with Strawberry Sauce, 272

Walnut Macaroons, 273

Apple Bread Pudding

~

Serve this pudding warm on those chilly winter nights!

NUTRITION FACTS
10 Servings
Serving Size 1/2 cup

AMOUNT PER SERVING

Exchanges
2 Starch

Calories	156	
Calories from Fat	12	
Total Fat	1	g
Saturated Fat	0	g
Cholesterol	2	mg
Sodium	218	mg
Total Carbohydrate	29	g
Dietary Fiber	3	g
Sugars	17	g
Protein	8	g

5–6 cups cubed whole-wheat bread (about 9 slices)
2 cups cubed apple (Granny Smith apples work well)
4 cups fat-free milk
1 cup egg substitute
2 tsp vanilla
2 tsp cinnamon
1/4 cup fructose
1/2 cup raisins

1. Preheat the oven to 350 degrees. In a large baking dish, combine the bread and apples.

2. In a separate bowl, whisk together the milk, egg substitute, vanilla, cinnamon, and fructose. Add the raisins. Pour the milk mixture over the bread and let stand for 15 minutes so the bread can absorb some of the liquid.

3. Bake for 40 to 45 minutes until the bread pudding is set and firm. Cut into squares and serve warm with whipped topping or low fat ice cream.

Apple Cranberry Crisp

This is a great holiday dessert!
It's good served with low-fat vanilla ice cream.

7 medium apples, cored and sliced
1 cup cranberries, chopped or
   left whole
2 Tbsp lemon juice
1 tsp cinnamon
1 tsp nutmeg

1/4 cup whole-wheat flour
1/2 cup rolled oats
2 Tbsp canola oil
2 Tbsp fructose
1 tsp vanilla

1. Preheat the oven to 325 degrees. Spray an 8 × 8 × 2-inch baking dish with nonstick cooking spray and layer the apples and cranberries in the dish.

2. Combine the lemon juice and spices in a small bowl; pour over the apples and cranberries.

3. Combine the flour, oats, oil, fructose, and vanilla and stir until the mixture looks like granola. Sprinkle over the apples and cranberries.

4. Bake the crisp uncovered for 20 minutes. Broil the top of the crisp for 2 minutes until the top is slightly browned, if desired.

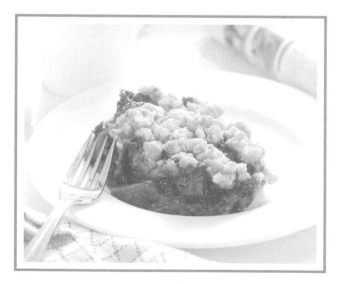

NUTRITION FACTS

8 Servings
Serving Size 1/2 cup

AMOUNT PER SERVING

Exchanges
1 Starch
1 Fruit
1 Fat

Calories	161
Calories from Fat	40
Total Fat	4 g
Saturated Fat	0 g
Cholesterol	0 mg
Sodium	1 mg
Total Carbohydrate	31 g
Dietary Fiber	5 g
Sugars	21 g
Protein	2 g

Banana Pineapple Freeze

Try this dessert when you are in the mood for something cool and creamy without all the fat of ice cream. It's especially pretty served in wine or champagne glasses and topped with a sprig of mint.

2 cups mashed ripe bananas
2 cups unsweetened orange juice
2 Tbsp fresh lemon juice

1 cup unsweetened crushed pineapple, undrained
Ground cinnamon

1. Combine all ingredients in a food processor, processing until smooth and creamy.
2. Pour mixture into a 9 × 9 × 2-inch baking dish and freeze overnight or until firm. Serve chilled.

Bananas Foster

This is a light version of a classic, elegant favorite.

1/2 cup unsweetened pineapple
   juice
1/4 tsp cinnamon
3 large bananas

1 cup unsweetened sliced
   pineapple, drained
1/4 cup rum
1 quart fat-free, no-sugar-added
   vanilla ice cream

1. In a medium skillet, combine the pineapple juice and cinnamon.
2. Peel the bananas and slice in half crosswise; quarter each piece
   lengthwise.
3. Add the bananas and pineapple slices to juice mixture and cook over
   medium heat until bananas are soft, basting constantly with juice.
4. Place rum in a small, long-handled skillet and heat until warm. Ignite
   the rum with a long match and quickly pour over the fruit.
5. Arrange ice cream in a serving dish, spoon bananas over the ice cream,
   and serve immediately.

NUTRITION FACTS

8 Servings
Serving Size 1/2 cup ice
  cream with 1/8 of the
  banana sauce

AMOUNT PER SERVING

Exchanges
2 1/2 Carbohydrate

Calories	159	
Calories from Fat	2	
Total Fat	0	g
Saturated Fat	0	g
Cholesterol	4	mg
Sodium	71	mg
Total Carbohydrate	37	g
Dietary Fiber	7	g
Sugars	16	g
Protein	5	g

Basic Crêpes

Any filling is great stuffed into these basic crêpes, depending on whether you're serving hearty main entrees or spectacular desserts!

3/4 cup egg substitute
1 1/3 cups flour
1/2 tsp salt

1 1/2 cups fat-free milk
2 tsp canola oil

1. Combine all ingredients in a food processor or blender. Process for 30 seconds, scraping down the sides of the container. Continue to process until mixture is smooth; refrigerate for 1 hour.

2. Coat the bottom of a 6-inch crêpe pan or small skillet with nonstick cooking spray. Place the pan over medium heat until hot but not smoking.

3. Pour 2 Tbsp of batter into the pan and quickly tilt it in all directions so that the batter covers the pan in a thin film. Cook for about 1 minute, lifting the edge of the crêpe to test for doneness (the crêpe is ready to be flipped when it can be shaken loose from the pan).

4. Flip the crêpe and continue to cook for 30 seconds on the other side. (This side usually has brownish spots on it, so place the filling on this side.)

5. Stack the cooked crêpes between layers of waxed paper to avoid sticking, and repeat the process with the remaining batter.

Basic Crêpes
with Fruit Filling

For these fruity dessert crêpes, select strawberries, blueberries, rasp-berries, or blackberries—or your own favorite fruit!

2 cups washed berries

1 cup water

2 tsp granulated sugar substitute

1 1/2 Tbsp cornstarch

20 Basic Crêpes (see recipe, page 247)

2 1/2 cups prepared Low-Calorie, Fat-Free Whipped Cream (see recipe, page 262)

1. Combine berries, water, sugar substitute, and cornstarch in a saucepan and bring to a boil. Lower heat until the mixture thickens.

2. Cool fruit mixture slightly; place mixture inside each of 20 crêpes. Fold the crêpe over to seal it. Top each crêpe with 2 Tbsp of the whipped cream topping.

NUTRITION FACTS

16 Servings
Serving Size 1 slice

AMOUNT PER SERVING

Exchanges
1 Starch
1 1/2 Fat

Calories	155
Calories from Fat	83
Total Fat	9 g
Saturated Fat	1 g
Cholesterol	0 mg
Sodium	106 mg
with added salt	173 mg
Total Carbohydrate	15 g
Dietary Fiber	1 g
Sugars	2 g
Protein	3 g

Carrot Cake

*Applesauce replaces some of the fat used in this
dense, moist cake to produce a delicious, good-for-you taste!*

1/2 cup canola oil

1/2 cup unsweetened applesauce

2 Tbsp granulated sugar substitute

1 cup egg substitute

1/2 cup water

2 cups flour

1 tsp baking powder

1 tsp baking soda

2 tsp cinnamon

1/4 tsp nutmeg

1/2 tsp salt (optional)

1/2 cup chopped pecans

3 cups grated carrots

1. Preheat the oven to 350 degrees. In a large mixing bowl, beat together the oil, applesauce, sugar substitute, and egg substitute until well blended.

2. Add the water, flour, baking powder, baking soda, cinnamon, nutmeg, and salt and mix well.

3. Stir in the pecans and carrots. Coat a 3-quart tube pan with nonstick cooking spray. Pour in the batter and bake for 35 to 40 minutes or until a toothpick inserted in the cake comes out clean.

4. Let the cake cool 10 minutes in the pan, then invert cake and let cool completely. If you like, frost with Low-Fat Cream Cheese Frosting (see recipe, page 263).

Cherry Cheesecake

You can substitute blueberries or strawberries for the cherries in this creamy cheesecake if you like.

12 oz evaporated fat-free milk

4 Tbsp cornstarch (divided use)

1/4 cup granulated sugar substitute

4 oz fat-free cream cheese, softened

2 oz reduced-fat cream cheese, softened

1/2 cup fresh lemon juice

1 tsp vanilla

1 prepared Crumb Pie Shell (see recipe, page 259, and omit cinnamon)

12 oz unsweetened sour cherries, undrained

1 Tbsp sugar substitute

1. In a saucepan over medium heat, whisk the milk and 2 Tbsp cornstarch constantly, but do not boil, until thickened. Remove from heat, stir in the sugar substitute, and set aside to cool.

2. In a small bowl, beat the cream cheese until light and fluffy. Add to cool milk mixture; beat in lemon juice and vanilla. Pour mixture into prepared pie shell and refrigerate overnight until firm.

3. To prepare the topping, drain the cherries over a saucepan so that only the liquid goes into the saucepan. Add 2 Tbsp cornstarch to the cherry liquid and simmer over medium heat until the mixture is thick and clear.

4. Stir in the cherries and sugar substitute, mixing thoroughly. Remove from heat and let cool. Spread topping over cheesecake and refrigerate until ready to serve.

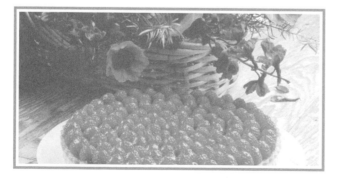

NUTRITION FACTS

10 Servings
Serving Size 1 slice

AMOUNT PER SERVING

Exchanges
1 1/2 Carbohydrate
1/2 Fat

Calories	149
Calories from Fat	36
Total Fat	4 g
Saturated Fat	1 g
Cholesterol	10 mg
Sodium	208 mg
Total Carbohydrate	21 g
Dietary Fiber	1 g
Sugars	9 g
Protein	7 g

Cherry Cobbler

You can find arrowroot powder in the spice aisle of the supermarket.

2 cups water-packed sour cherries
1/4 tsp fresh lemon juice
1/8 tsp almond extract
1/2 tsp arrowroot powder
1/2 cup flour, sifted
1/8 tsp salt (optional)

3/4 tsp baking powder
1 Tbsp reduced-fat margarine
1/4 cup egg substitute
2 Tbsp fat-free milk
1/4 cup granulated sugar substitute

1. Preheat the oven to 425 degrees. Drain cherries, reserving 2/3 cup of liquid, and place the cherries in a shallow cake pan.

2. In a small mixing bowl, combine the lemon juice, almond extract, arrowroot powder, and drained cherry liquid; mix well. Spoon over the cherries.

3. In a mixing bowl, combine the flour, salt, and baking powder. Mix thoroughly. Cut in margarine until coarse; add egg substitute, milk, and sugar substitute, mixing well.

4. Spoon mixture over cherries and bake for 25 to 30 minutes or until crust is golden brown.

Cherry Pie

This is a beautiful pie to make for company or Valentine's Day, with heart-shaped cutouts and warm red cherries!

32 oz water-packed sour cherries, undrained

3 Tbsp cornstarch

1/4 cup granulated sugar substitute

1/4 tsp almond extract

Red food coloring (optional)

1 prepared Graham Kerr's Basic Pie Crust, unbaked (see recipe, page 261—be sure to read step 3 of this cherry pie recipe before rolling out the pie crust dough!)

1. Preheat the oven to 425 degrees. Drain cherries; reserve 1/2 cup of the juice.

2. In a large saucepan, combine the cherry juice, cornstarch, sugar substitute, and almond extract. Let the mixture simmer over medium heat until slightly thickened. (If you like, add a few drops of red food coloring to achieve a more intense color.) Fold in the cherries and set aside.

3. Roll out the pie dough on a lightly floured surface into a circle larger than a 9-inch pie plate. Place the dough into the pie plate, securing it by pressing the edges with the tines of a fork. Cut away the excess dough and roll it out very thin. Cut out 8 heart-shaped designs with a cookie cutter; prick the sides and bottom of shell with a fork.

4. Pour cherry filling into pie shell, and arrange hearts evenly around the top. Bake for 40 to 50 minutes or until crust is lightly browned. If you like, serve with Low-Calorie, Fat-Free Whipped Cream (see recipe, page 262) or low-fat ice cream.

NUTRITION FACTS

8 Servings
Serving Size 1 slice

AMOUNT PER SERVING

Exchanges
2 Carbohydrate
1/2 Fat

Calories	159
Calories from Fat	37
Total Fat	4 g
Saturated Fat	1 g
Cholesterol	0 mg
Sodium	54 mg
Total Carbohydrate	29 g
Dietary Fiber	1 g
Sugars	12 g
Protein	2 g

Cherry Soufflé

*Try this soufflé when you want something different
from a traditional pie.*

3/4 cup water
1 package unflavored gelatin
2 cups water-packed sour cherries,
 drained and chopped
1 Tbsp fresh lemon juice

2 Tbsp granulated sugar substitute
3 large egg whites
2 cups prepared Low-Calorie,
 Fat-Free Whipped Cream
 (see recipe, page 262)

1. In a medium saucepan, combine the water and gelatin; allow to soften
 for 10 to 15 minutes. Add 1 cup of the cherries, lemon juice, and sugar
 substitute; bring to a boil.

2. Remove from heat and let cool; refrigerate until thick and syrupy.

3. Fold in remaining cherries, beaten egg whites, and whipped cream.
 Spoon into a soufflé dish and refrigerate until set.

NUTRITION FACTS

8 Servings
Serving Size 1/8 soufflé

AMOUNT PER SERVING

Exchanges
1 Starch

Calories	68
Calories from Fat	0
Total Fat	0 g
Saturated Fat	0 g
Cholesterol	2 mg
Sodium	68 mg
Total Carbohydrate	11 g
Dietary Fiber	1 g
Sugars	10 g
Protein	6 g

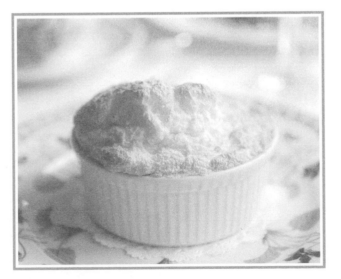

Chocolate Chip Cookies

This version of chocolate chip cookies has a delicious cake-like texture.

1/4 cup reduced-fat margarine
2 Tbsp granulated sugar substitute
2 Tbsp brown sugar substitute
1/4 cup egg substitute
3 Tbsp water
1 tsp vanilla

3/4 cup flour
1/4 tsp baking soda
1/4 tsp salt
6 Tbsp semisweet chocolate mini
   morsels

1. Preheat the oven to 375 degrees. In a medium bowl, cream the margarine and the sugar substitutes. Beat in the egg substitute, water, and vanilla; mix thoroughly.

2. In a sifter, combine the flour, baking soda, and salt. Sift the dry ingredients into the creamed mixture and mix well. Stir in the chocolate mini morsels.

3. Lightly spray cookie sheets with nonstick cooking spray. Drop teaspoonfuls of dough onto cookie sheets and bake for 8 to 10 minutes. Remove the cookies from the oven and cool them on racks.

NUTRITION FACTS
15 Servings
Serving Size 2 cookies

AMOUNT PER SERVING

Exchanges
1/2 Carbohydrate
1 Fat

Calories	69	
Calories from Fat	32	
Total Fat	4	g
Saturated Fat	1	g
Cholesterol	0	mg
Sodium	94	mg
Total Carbohydrate	8	g
Dietary Fiber	0	g
Sugars	3	g
Protein	1	g

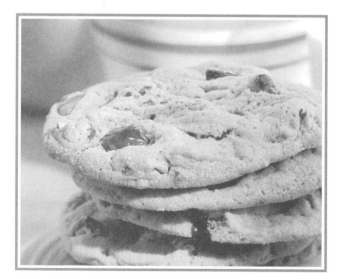

Chocolate Cupcakes

A healthier version of everyone's favorite! Try frosting these with Low-Fat Cream Cheese Frosting (see recipe, page 263).

2 Tbsp reduced-fat margarine
2 Tbsp canola oil
1/4 cup fructose
1/4 cup egg substitute
1 tsp vanilla
1/2 cup fat-free milk

1 1/4 cups flour
1/4 cup ground walnuts
6 Tbsp cocoa powder
2 tsp baking powder
1/4 tsp baking soda

1. Preheat the oven to 375 degrees. Beat the margarine with the oil until creamy. Add the fructose, then egg substitute, vanilla, and milk.

2. In a separate bowl, combine the flour, walnuts, cocoa, baking powder, and baking soda. Add to the creamed mixture and mix until smooth.

3. Spoon the batter into paper-lined muffin tins and bake for 20 minutes. Remove from the oven and let cool.

Chocolate Rum Pie

Just a hint of rum complements the chocolate in this elegant dessert.

1 package unflavored gelatin
1 cup fat-free milk
2 eggs, separated
2 Tbsp granulated sugar substitute
1/4 cup cocoa
1 tsp rum extract

1 Tbsp liquid sugar substitute
2 cups fat-free whipped topping
1 prepared Graham Kerr's Basic
   Pie Crust, baked (see recipe,
   page 261)

1. In a large saucepan, combine gelatin, milk, egg yolks, granulated sugar substitute, and cocoa. Cook over medium heat until completely blended and slightly thickened.
2. Remove from heat, stir in the rum extract, and refrigerate the mixture until partially set.
3. In a small bowl, beat egg whites with liquid sugar substitute until stiff peaks form. Fold into cooled chocolate mixture.
4. Layer the chocolate mixture and whipped topping in the pie shell, ending with whipped topping. Refrigerate for 2 to 3 hours or until firm.

NUTRITION FACTS
8 Servings
Serving Size 1 slice

AMOUNT PER SERVING

Exchanges
1 1/2 Carbohydrate
1 Fat

Calories	154	
Calories from Fat	51	
Total Fat	6	g
Saturated Fat	1	g
Cholesterol	53	mg
Sodium	89	mg
Total Carbohydrate	20	g
Dietary Fiber	1	g
Sugars	5	g
Protein	5	g

Cream Cheese Cookies

You can freeze the rolled dough for these cookies (after step 2), pull it out when you need it, and make warm cookies fast for holidays or special occasions!

1/4 cup vegetable shortening
2 oz low-fat cream cheese, softened
1 Tbsp fructose
1/4 cup egg substitute

1 Tbsp water
1 cup flour
1/2 tsp baking powder
Dash salt (optional)

1. In a food processor, combine shortening, cream cheese, and fructose; mix until creamy in texture. Add the egg substitute and water; mix thoroughly.

2. Sift flour, baking powder, and salt (if desired) together and add to creamed mixture; blend well. Shape into a roll about 1 1/2 inches in diameter and refrigerate overnight.

3. Preheat the oven to 350 degrees. Cut dough into 1 1/2-inch slices and place on ungreased cookie sheets.

4. Bake cookies for 8 to 10 minutes or until the tops are golden brown. Remove cookies from the oven and let them cool on racks.

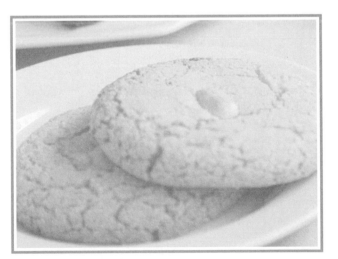

Crêpes Suzette

Now you can make this classic French recipe—always dramatic to serve!

2 cups unsweetened orange juice
2 Tbsp cornstarch
1 Tbsp orange rind
2 medium oranges, peeled and
    sectioned

16 Basic Crêpes (see recipe, page
    247)
1/4 cup Grand Marnier

1. In a large skillet, combine the orange juice, cornstarch, and orange rind. Bring the mixture to a boil over medium heat. Boil for 1 to 2 minutes, stirring occasionally.

2. Add the orange sections and remove from heat. Allow the mixture to cool slightly.

3. Dip both sides of the crêpes in sauce; fold in quarters. Arrange crêpes in the skillet in the remaining sauce; heat completely over low heat.

4. Heat (do not boil!) Grand Marnier in a saucepan over medium heat, then ignite it with a long match and pour over the crêpes. Serve when the flame subsides.

NUTRITION FACTS
8 Servings
Serving Size 2 crêpes

AMOUNT PER SERVING

Exchanges
2 Starch

Calories	156
Calories from Fat	11
Total Fat	1 g
Saturated Fat	0 g
Cholesterol	1 mg
Sodium	151 mg
Total Carbohydrate	31 g
Dietary Fiber	1 g
Sugars	16 g
Protein	5 g

Crumb Pie Shell

~

You can use this basic pie shell with almost any filling.

1 1/4 cups finely crumbled Zwie-
back crackers

3 Tbsp reduced-fat margarine,
melted

1 Tbsp water

1/8 tsp cinnamon

1. Preheat the oven to 325 degrees. In a medium mixing bowl, combine the cracker crumbs, margarine, water, and cinnamon, mixing thoroughly.

2. Spread the mixture evenly into a 10-inch pie pan. Press the mixture firmly onto the sides and bottom of the pan.

3. Bake the pie shell for 8 to 10 minutes. You can refrigerate it after baking until ready to use.

Fresh Apple Pie

*You can substitute peaches or berries for the apples
in this delicious homemade pie.*

10 medium baking apples (Rome
   apples work well), peeled, cored,
   and sliced (3 lb total)
2 tsp fresh lemon juice
1 prepared Graham Kerr's Basic
   Pie Crust, unbaked (see recipe,
   page 261)

2 Tbsp granulated sugar substitute
1 Tbsp flour
1 tsp ground cinnamon
1/2 tsp ground nutmeg

1. Preheat the oven to 425 degrees. Place the sliced apples in a large bowl,
   sprinkle with lemon juice, and toss to coat. Arrange the apples in the pie
   shell.

2. In a small bowl, combine the sugar substitute, flour, cinnamon, and
   nutmeg; mix well. Sprinkle the mixture over the apples.

3. Cover the edges of the crust with foil so they don't burn. Bake the pie for
   35 to 40 minutes or until the crust is golden brown. Remove from the
   oven and cool slightly before serving.

NUTRITION FACTS

8 Servings
Serving Size 1 slice

AMOUNT PER SERVING

Exchanges
2 1/2 Carbohydrate
1/2 Fat

Calories	183	
Calories from Fat	41	
Total Fat	5	g
Saturated Fat	1	g
Cholesterol	0	mg
Sodium	46	mg
Total Carbohydrate	36	g
Dietary Fiber	3	g
Sugars	23	g
Protein	1	g

NUTRITION FACTS

8 Servings
Serving Size 1/8 shell

AMOUNT PER SERVING

Exchanges
1/2 Starch
1 Fat

Calories	82
Calories from Fat	36
Total Fat	4 g
Saturated Fat	1 g
Cholesterol	0 mg
Sodium	45 mg
Total Carbohydrate	10 g
Dietary Fiber	0 g
Sugars	0 g
Protein	1 g

Graham Kerr's Basic Pie Crust

Graham Kerr developed this tasty, low-fat alternative to the classic pie shell recipe. You can use this recipe for an 8- or 9-inch pie crust.

3/4 cup cake flour
1/2 tsp sugar
Pinch salt
1 Tbsp non-aromatic olive oil

2 Tbsp hard margarine (65% vegetable type), frozen for 15 minutes
1/2 tsp vinegar
2 Tbsp ice water

1. In a medium bowl, combine the flour, sugar, and salt. Stir in the oil. Add the margarine and cut in with a pastry cutter until the mixture is the size of small peas.

2. Add the vinegar and ice water and mix with a fork until the dough starts to hold together. Gather into a ball, wrap, and refrigerate at least 30 minutes before rolling out.

3. Roll out the pie crust to fit an 8- or 9-inch pie dish. Lay rolled dough in the pan without stretching it, and crimp the edges.

4. If the recipe requires a baked pie crust, preheat the oven to 425 degrees. Prick the crust with a fork, and lay a piece of parchment or waxed paper in the pie shell. Pour in enough dried beans to cover the bottom (this prevents the crust from bubbling up while baking). Bake for 8 minutes or until golden brown.

Low-Calorie, Fat-Free Whipped Cream

Use this delicious whipped cream topping on fruit, pies, or cakes.

2 Tbsp water
1 tsp unflavored gelatin
1/2 cup fat-free powdered milk

1 tsp vanilla extract
1 cup ice water
1/2 tsp liquid sugar substitute

1. In a small skillet, add the water; sprinkle gelatin on top.

2. After the gelatin has soaked in, stir over low heat until clear; cool. In a large mixing bowl, combine the milk, vanilla, ice water, and sugar substitute; mix well.

3. Add the gelatin mixture and whip until fluffy with a wire whisk or electric beaters. Refrigerate whipped cream until ready to use.

NUTRITION FACTS
8 Servings
Serving Size 2 Tbsp

AMOUNT PER SERVING

Exchanges
Free Food*

Calories	16
Calories from Fat	0
Total Fat	0 g
Saturated Fat	0 g
Cholesterol	1 mg
Sodium	25 mg
Total Carbohydrate	2 g
Dietary Fiber	0 g
Sugars	2 g
Protein	2 g

*Remember that only 2 Tbsp or less is a Free Food!

NUTRITION FACTS

48 Servings
Serving Size 2 Tbsp

AMOUNT PER SERVING

Exchanges
1/2 Fat-Free Milk

Calories	38
Calories from Fat	13
Total Fat	1 g
Saturated Fat	1 g
Cholesterol	6 mg
Sodium	63 mg
Total Carbohydrate	3 g
Dietary Fiber	0 g
Sugars	2 g
Protein	3 g

Low-Fat Cream Cheese Frosting

This is a delicious, low-fat version of an old favorite!

3 cups fat-free ricotta cheese

1 1/3 cups plain fat-free yogurt, strained overnight in cheesecloth over a bowl set in the refrigerator

2 cups low-fat cottage cheese

1/3 cup fructose

3 Tbsp evaporated fat-free milk

1. Combine all the ingredients in a large bowl; beat well with electric beaters until slightly stiff.

2. Place frosting in a covered container and refrigerate until ready to use (this frosting can be refrigerated for up to 1 week).

Oatmeal Raisin Cookies

Whole-wheat flour and oats add fiber to these tasty cookies.

3 cups rolled oats

1 cup whole-wheat flour

1 tsp baking soda

2 tsp cinnamon

1/2 cup raisins

1/4 cup unsweetened applesauce

1/4 cup fructose

1/2 cup egg substitute

1/2 cup plain fat-free yogurt

1 tsp vanilla

1. Preheat the oven to 350 degrees. Combine the oats, flour, baking soda, cinnamon, and raisins.

2. Beat the applesauce, fructose, egg substitute, yogurt, and vanilla in a large bowl until creamy. Slowly add the dry ingredients and mix together.

3. Spray cookie sheets with nonstick cooking spray and drop by teaspoonfuls onto the cookie sheets. Bake for 12 to 15 minutes; transfer to racks and cool.

NUTRITION FACTS

24 Servings
Serving Size 2 cookies

AMOUNT PER SERVING

Exchanges
1 Starch

Calories	76	
Calories from Fat	7	
Total Fat	1	g
Saturated Fat	0	g
Cholesterol	0	mg
Sodium	46	mg
Total Carbohydrate	15	g
Dietary Fiber	2	g
Sugars	4	g
Protein	3	g

Peach Crumb Cobbler

*If you like, you can substitute pears, apples, or berries
for the peaches in this tasty cobbler.*

2 cups fresh peaches, sliced
1/3 cup graham cracker crumbs
1/2 tsp ground cinnamon

1/4 tsp nutmeg
2 tsp reduced-fat margarine

1. Preheat the oven to 350 degrees. Place the sliced peaches in the bottom of an 8 × 8 × 2-inch baking pan. In a small mixing bowl, combine the graham cracker crumbs, cinnamon, and nutmeg; mix well.
2. Gradually blend in margarine and sprinkle mixture over peaches. Bake uncovered for 25 to 30 minutes. Remove from oven and let cool slightly before serving.

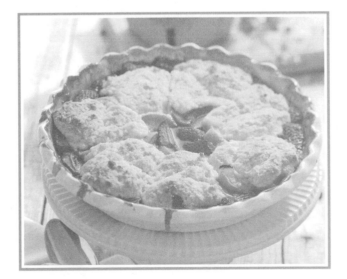

Peach Shortcake

This is a perfect summer dessert—fresh peaches over a tender cake crust.

2 cups sliced fresh peaches
1 1/2 Tbsp plus 1 tsp granulated
   sugar substitute
1/2 tsp almond extract
1/2 tsp cinnamon
1 cup flour

2 tsp baking powder
Dash salt (optional)
2 Tbsp canola oil
1/4 cup egg substitute
1/4 cup fat-free milk

1. Preheat the oven to 400 degrees. Lightly spray an 8 × 8 × 2-inch baking pan with nonstick cooking spray. Arrange the peaches in the bottom of the dish.

2. Mix together 1 tsp sugar substitute, almond extract, and cinnamon; sprinkle over the peaches and set aside. In a medium mixing bowl, combine the flour, baking powder, salt, and 1 1/2 Tbsp sugar substitute; mix well.

3. Add the oil, egg substitute, and milk to the dry ingredients; mix until smooth. Spread evenly over the peaches and bake for 25 to 30 minutes or until the top is golden brown. Remove from oven, invert onto a serving plate, and serve.

NUTRITION FACTS
8 Servings
Serving Size 1/2 cup

AMOUNT PER SERVING

Exchanges
1 Starch
1/2 Fruit

Calories	114	
Calories from Fat	33	
Total Fat	4	g
Saturated Fat	0	g
Cholesterol	0	mg
Sodium	94	mg
with added salt	110	mg
Total Carbohydrate	18	g
Dietary Fiber	1	g
Sugars	5	g
Protein	3	g

Peanut Butter Cookies

Note that these cookies require overnight refrigeration before baking.

1/4 cup reduced-fat margarine
1/4 cup creamy peanut butter
2 Tbsp brown sugar substitute
1/4 cup egg substitute
1/4 cup water

1 tsp vanilla
1 1/2 cups flour
1 tsp baking soda
1/2 tsp baking powder

1. Preheat the oven to 375 degrees.

2. In a food processor or by hand, cream together the margarine, peanut butter, and sugar substitute. Add the egg substitute, water, and vanilla and continue to mix until well blended.

2. Combine the flour, baking soda, and baking powder in a sifter; sift dry ingredients into creamed mixture and mix until completely blended. Refrigerate overnight.

3. Lightly spray cookie sheets with nonstick cooking spray. Drop teaspoonfuls onto cookie sheets and press with the tines of a fork to flatten each cookie.

4. Bake the cookies for 12 to 15 minutes, remove from the oven, and let them cool on racks.

Pineapple Pear Medley

Cooking the fruit juices and then allowing the dish to cool in the refrigerator creates a unique, refreshing flavor.

1 large orange
1 15-oz can unsweetened pineapple chunks, undrained
32 oz unsweetened pear halves, drained

1 16-oz can unsweetened apricot halves, drained
6 whole cloves
2 cinnamon sticks

1. Peel the orange and reserve the rind. Divide the orange into sections and remove the membrane.

2. Drain the pineapple, reserve the juice, and set aside. In a large bowl, combine the orange sections, pineapple, pears, and apricots. Toss and set aside.

3. In a small saucepan over medium heat, combine orange rind, pineapple juice, cloves, and cinnamon. Let simmer for 5 to 10 minutes, then strain the juices and pour over the fruit.

4. Cover and refrigerate for at least 2 to 3 hours. Toss before serving.

NUTRITION FACTS

12 Servings
Serving Size 1/2 cup

AMOUNT PER SERVING

Exchanges
1 Fruit

Calories	50
Calories from Fat	0
Total Fat	0 g
Saturated Fat	0 g
Cholesterol	0 mg
Sodium	3 mg
Total Carbohydrate	13 g
Dietary Fiber	3 g
Sugars	10 g
Protein	1 g

NUTRITION FACTS

4 Servings
Serving Size 1/2 cup

AMOUNT PER SERVING

Exchanges
1/2 Starch

Calories	61	
Calories from Fat	0	
Total Fat	0	g
Saturated Fat	0	g
Cholesterol	2	mg
Sodium	72	mg
Total Carbohydrate	9	g
Dietary Fiber	1	g
Sugars	8	g
Protein	6	g

Pumpkin Mousse

~

This is a perfect addition to your Thanksgiving buffet table.

1 package unflavored gelatin
1/2 cup water
2/3 cup instant fat-free milk powder
1/2 cup mashed pumpkin

2 Tbsp granulated sugar substitute
1/2 tsp vanilla extract
1 tsp pumpkin pie spice
6 ice cubes

1. Combine the gelatin and water in a small saucepan and let stand for 1 to 2 minutes. Place over medium heat, stirring constantly, for 1 to 2 minutes or until gelatin is dissolved.

2. Combine the gelatin, milk powder, pumpkin, sugar substitute, vanilla, and pumpkin pie spice in blender or food processor; process until very smooth. Add ice cubes to the mixture, one at a time, blending thoroughly after each addition.

3. Pour into 4 parfait glasses or dessert dishes, cover, and refrigerate for 2 to 3 hours before serving. Top with Low-Caloric, Fat-Free Whipped Cream if desired (see recipe, page 262).

Sponge Cake

*Try topping this light sponge cake with fresh fruit and
Low-Calorie, Fat-Free Whipped Cream (see recipe, page 262), and
you'll have a delicious summer dessert!*

4 large eggs, separated
3 Tbsp granulated sugar substitute
1/2 cup hot water
1 1/2 tsp vanilla extract

1 1/2 cups cake flour, sifted
1/4 tsp salt
1/4 tsp baking powder

1. Preheat the oven to 325 degrees. In a medium bowl, beat egg yolks
   and sugar substitute until thick and lemon-colored. Add the hot water
   and vanilla and continue beating for 3 more minutes.

2. In a sifter, combine flour, salt, and baking powder; add to the egg yolk
   mixture.

3. Beat the egg whites until stiff and fold into egg yolk mixture. Spoon batter into an ungreased 9-inch tube pan and bake for 50 to 60 minutes or
   until a toothpick inserted comes out clean.

4. Remove the cake from the oven and invert it onto a plate. Allow the cake
   to sit inverted in its pan for at least 1 hour. Remove the pan and let cake
   cool completely.

NUTRITION FACTS

12 Servings
Serving Size 1 slice

AMOUNT PER SERVING

Exchanges
1 Starch

Calories	76	
Calories from Fat	16	
Total Fat	2	g
Saturated Fat	1	g
Cholesterol	71	mg
Sodium	74	mg
Total Carbohydrate	11	g
Dietary Fiber	0	g
Sugars	1	g
Protein	3	g

Strawberries Romanoff

The low-fat versions of ice cream and whipped cream make this recipe healthy and delicious!

2 cups fresh strawberries, hulled
1 cup low-fat vanilla ice cream
1 Tbsp orange marmalade
1 tsp rum extract

1/2 cup prepared Low-Calorie, Fat-Free Whipped Cream (see recipe, page 262)

1. Divide strawberries evenly between 4 serving dishes and refrigerate.
2. Just before serving, fold ice cream, orange marmalade, rum extract, and whipped cream together in a medium bowl. Spoon evenly over chilled strawberries and serve.

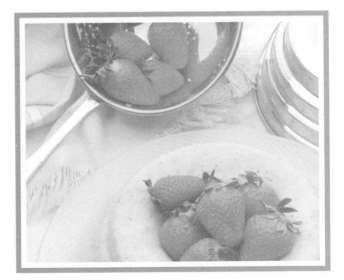

Strawberries with Strawberry Sauce

Strawberry fans will love this easy, fast dessert!

4 cups fresh strawberries, washed and stemmed

1 tsp sugar substitute

2 Tbsp fresh orange juice

1/2 cup fresh blueberries for topping

1. Divide 2 cups of strawberries among 6 dessert dishes.
2. Puree the remaining 2 cups of strawberries in a blender with the sugar substitute and orange juice. Pour the sauce evenly over the dessert cups. Top each dessert cup with blueberries.

NUTRITION FACTS

6 Servings
Serving Size 1/2 cup

AMOUNT PER SERVING

Exchanges
1/2 Fruit

Calories	41	
Calories from Fat	0	
Total Fat	0	g
Saturated Fat	0	g
Cholesterol	0	mg
Sodium	2	mg
Total Carbohydrate	10	g
Dietary Fiber	3	g
Sugars	6	g
Protein	1	g

Walnut Macaroons

Note that you'll need to refrigerate this cookie dough overnight.

2 cups quick-cooking oats
2 Tbsp granulated sugar substitute
1/4 tsp salt (optional)
2 tsp vanilla

1/2 cup canola oil
1/4 cup egg substitute, beaten
1/2 cup finely chopped walnuts

1. In a medium bowl, combine the oats, sugar substitute, salt, vanilla, and oil; mix thoroughly. Cover and refrigerate overnight.
2. Preheat the oven to 350 degrees. Add egg substitute and walnuts to mixture; blend thoroughly.
3. Pack cookie mixture into a teaspoon, level, and push out onto ungreased cookie sheets.
4. Bake cookies for 15 minutes or until tops are golden brown. Transfer cookies to racks and cool.

Index

Appetizers (*also see* Dips)
Baked Scallops, 3
Broiled Shrimp with Garlic, 4
Cheesy Tortilla Wedges, 5
Cherry Tomatoes Stuffed with Crab, 6
Chicken Kabobs, 7
Chilled Shrimp, 8
Crab Cakes, 9
Crab-Filled Mushrooms, 10
Cucumber Paté, 12
Monterey Jack Cheese Quiche Squares, 20
Stuffed Shrimp, 21
Turkey Meatballs, 22

Beans
Black Bean Salad, 37
Spanish Black Bean Soup, 78
White Bean Soup, 80

Beef (*also see* Veal)
Baked Steak with Creole Sauce, 134
Beef Provençal, 135
Beef Shish Kabobs, 136
Beef Stroganoff, 84
Butterflied Beef Eye Roast, 137
Herbed Pot Roast, 138
Marinated Beef Kabobs, 142
Marvelous Meat Loaf, 144

Roast Beef with Caraway Seeds, 147
Steak with Brandied Onions, 148
Stuffed Bell Peppers, 150

Breads (*also see* Muffins)
Blueberry Scones, 218
Buttermilk Biscuits, 219
Cranberry Orange Scones, 221
Date Nut Bread, 222
Homemade Seasoned Bread
    Crumbs, 223
Irish Soda Bread, 224
Spoon Bread, 226
Sweet Potato and Zucchini Bread, 227

Breakfasts
Baked French Toast with Raspberry
    Sauce, 231
Fresh Blueberry Pancakes, 232
Fruit Puff Pancake, 233
Griddle Corn Cakes, 234
Hash Browns, 235
Italian Frittata, 236
Mini Breakfast Quiches, 237
Turkey Sausage Patties, 238
Western Omelet, 239

Cheese
Baked Macaroni and Cheese, 83
Cheesy Tortilla Wedges, 5
Cherry Cheesecake, 250
Cream Cheese Cookies, 257
Green Bean, Walnut, and Feta Salad, 44
Gruyere Apple Spread, 14
Low-Fat Cream Cheese Frosting, 263
Monterey Jack Cheese Quiche Squares, 20
Tortellini and Feta Cheese Salad, 55

Chicken Main Dishes
Baked Chicken and Peas, 102
Baked Chicken Breasts Supreme, 103
Baked Chicken Kiev, 104
Baked Chicken with Wine Sauce, 105
Baked Lemon Chicken, 106
Chicken and Shrimp, 107
Chicken and Zucchini, 108
Chicken Dijon, 109
Chicken Paprika, 110
Chicken Parmesan, 111
Chicken Provençal, 112
Chicken Rose Marie, 113
Chicken with Cream Sauce, 114
Chicken with Green Peppercorn
    Sauce, 115
Grilled Chicken with Garlic, 116
Grilled Lemon Mustard Chicken, 117
Marinated Chicken Kabobs, 120
Mushroom Chicken, 121
Oven-Baked Chicken Tenders, 122
Poached Chicken with Bay Leaves, 123
Sautéed Chicken with Artichoke
    Hearts, 124
Spicy Chicken Drumsticks, 125
Summer Chicken Kabobs, 126

Chicken Salads
Chinese Chicken Salad, 39
Mediterranean Chicken Salad, 48

Chicken Soup
Chicken and Mushroom Soup, 61
Chicken Stew with Noodles, 62

Chocolate
Chocolate Chip Cookies, 254

Chocolate Cupcakes, 255
Chocolate Rum Pie, 256

Clams
Linguine with Clam Sauce, 90
Pasta with Vegetable Clam Sauce, 92
Quick Manhattan Clam Chowder, 76

Crab
Crab and Rice Salad, 41
Crab Cakes, 9
Crab Imperial, 163
Crab-Filled Mushrooms, 10
Crabmeat Stuffing, 164
Hot Crab Dip, 17

Dips
Creamy Tarragon Dip, 11
Fresh Dill Dip, 13
Gruyere Apple Spread, 14
Guacamole, 15
Hot Artichoke Dip, 16
Hot Crab Dip, 17
Hummus, 18
Low-Fat Cream Cheese Dip, 19

Desserts (*also see* Fruit Desserts)
Basic Crêpes, 247
Carrot Cake, 249
Chocolate Chip Cookies, 254
Chocolate Cupcakes, 255
Chocolate Rum Pie, 256
Cream Cheese Cookies, 257
Crêpes Suzette, 258
Crumb Pie Shell, 259
Graham Kerr's Basic Pie Crust, 261
Low-Calorie, Fat-Free Whipped Cream, 262

Low-Fat Cream Cheese Frosting, 263
Oatmeal Raisin Cookies, 264
Peanut Butter Cookies, 267
Pumpkin Mousse, 269
Sponge Cake, 270
Walnut Macaroons, 273

Dressings & Sauces
Basic Barbecue Sauce, 25
Basic Vinaigrette, 26
Creamy Herb Dressing, 27
Dill Dressing, 28
French Dressing, 29
Ginger-Soy Dressing, 30
Marinara Sauce, 31
Mock Hollandaise, 32
Parmesan Dressing, 33
Tangy Marinade, 34

Fruit Desserts (*see* Desserts)
Apple Bread Pudding, 243
Apple Cranberry Crisp, 244
Banana Pineapple Freeze, 245
Bananas Foster, 246
Basic Crêpes with Fruit Filling, 248
Cherry Cheesecake, 250
Cherry Cobbler, 251
Cherry Pie, 252
Cherry Soufflé, 253
Fresh Apple Pie, 260
Peach Crumb Cobbler, 265
Peach Shortcake, 266
Pineapple Pear Medley, 268
Strawberries Romanoff, 271
Strawberries with Strawberry
    Sauce, 272

Game Hens
Apple-Glazed Cornish Hens, 101
Herbed Cornish Hens, 118

Lamb
Lamb Chops with Orange Sauce, 140
Lamb Kabobs, 141
Marinated Leg of Lamb, 143

Lentils
Lentil Salad, 46
Lentil Soup, 70

Muffins
Banana Carrot Muffins, 217
Corn Muffins, 220
Pineapple Muffins, 225

Mushrooms
Baked Shrimp and Mushroom
    Casserole, 160
Chicken and Mushroom Soup, 61
Crab-Filled Mushrooms, 10
Mushroom and Barley Soup, 72
Mushroom Cassoulets, 193
Mushroom Chicken, 121

Pasta
Baked Macaroni and Cheese, 83
Beef Stroganoff, 84
Corkscrew Pasta with Sage and
    Peppers, 85
Eggplant Lasagna, 86
Fettucine Verde with Tomato Sauce, 87
Fettucine with Peppers and Broccoli, 88
Garlic Fettucine, 89
Linguine with Clam Sauce, 90

Linguine with Garlic Broccoli Sauce, 91
Pasta with Vegetable Clam Sauce, 92
Rigatoni with Chicken and Three-
    Pepper Sauce, 93
Shrimp and Pasta Salad, 52
Spaghetti Pie, 94
Spaghetti with Pesto Sauce, 95
Stuffed Manicotti, 96
Vegetable Lo Mein, 97

Peppers
Corkscrew Pasta with Sage and
    Peppers, 85
Fettucine with Peppers and Broccoli, 88
Rigatoni with Chicken and Three-
    Pepper Sauce, 93
Sautéed Sweet Peppers, 194
Sherried Peppers with Bean Sprouts, 195
Stuffed Bell Peppers, 150

Pork
Apple Cinnamon Pork Chops, 133
Italian Pork Chops, 139
Pork Chops Milanese, 145
Pork Niçoise, 146
Stir-Fried Pork Tenderloin, 149

Potatoes
Baked Potato Toppers, 206
Festive Sweet Potatoes, 209
Greek Potato Salad, 43
Hash Browns, 235
Italian Potato Salad, 45
Potato Chowder, 75
Potato Parmesan Chips, 210
Sage Potatoes, 213
Scalloped Potatoes, 214

Poultry (*see* Chicken; Game Hens; Turkey)

Rice
Asian Fried Rice, 205
Colorful Rice Casserole, 207
Crab and Rice Salad, 41
Curried Rice with Pineapple, 208
Rice Parmesan, 211
Rice with Spinach and Feta, 212
Wild Rice Salad, 56

Salads
Black Bean Salad, 37
California Seafood Salad, 38
Chinese Chicken Salad, 39
Couscous Salad, 40
Crab and Rice Salad, 41
Fresh Seafood Pasta Salad, 42
Greek Potato Salad, 43
Green Bean, Walnut, and
    Feta Salad, 44
Italian Potato Salad, 45
Lentil Salad, 46
Lobster Salad, 47
Mediterranean Chicken Salad, 48
Overnight Coleslaw, 49
Pasta Salad–Stuffed Tomatoes, 50
Shanghai Salad, 51
Shrimp and Pasta Salad, 52
Shrimp and Radicchio Salad, 53
Tabbouleh Salad, 54
Tortellini and Feta Cheese Salad, 55
Wild Rice Salad, 56
Zucchini and Carrot Salad, 57

Sauces (*see* Dressings)

Seafood (*also see* Crab; Shrimp)
Baked Fish in Foil, 157
Broiled Sole with Mustard Sauce, 162
Fish Fillets with Tomatoes, 165
Flounder Parmesan, 166
Fresh Flounder Creole, 167
Grilled Salmon with Dill Sauce, 168
Grilled Scallop Kabobs, 169
Grilled Shark, 170
Grilled Swordfish with Rosemary, 171
Halibut Supreme, 172
Lobster Fricassee, 173
Pan-Fried Scallops, 174
Poached Red Snapper, 175
Sea Bass with Ginger Sauce, 176
Trout Amandine, 179
Vegetable Salmon Cakes, 180

Shrimp
Baked Garlic Scampi, 158
Baked Shrimp, 159
Baked Shrimp and Mushroom
    Casserole, 160
Basic Boiled Shrimp, 161
Broiled Shrimp with Garlic, 4
Chicken and Shrimp, 107
Chilled Shrimp, 8
Quick Shrimp Gumbo, 77
Shrimp and Pasta Salad, 52
Shrimp and Radicchio Salad, 53
Shrimp Creole, 177
Shrimp Provençal, 178
Stuffed Shrimp, 21

Soups & Stews
Chicken and Mushroom Soup, 61
Chicken Stew with Noodles, 62

Cream of Carrot Soup, 63
English Beef Stew, 64
French Onion Soup, 65
Fresh Fish Chowder, 66
Gazpacho, 67
Hearty Vegetable Soup, 68
Italian Minestrone, 69
Lentil Soup, 70
Mexican Tortilla Soup, 71
Mushroom and Barley Soup, 72
Old-Fashioned Vegetable Beef Stew, 73
Pasta Fagioli, 74
Potato Chowder, 75
Quick Manhattan Clam Chowder, 76
Quick Shrimp Gumbo, 77
Spanish Black Bean Soup, 78
Spicy Turkey Chili, 79
White Bean Soup, 80

Squash
Chicken and Zucchini, 108
Pumpkin Mousse, 169
Squash and Tomato Cassoulet, 197
Sweet Potato and Zucchini Bread, 227
Vegetable-Stuffed Yellow Squash, 200
Zucchini and Carrot Salad, 57
Zucchini and Onion Kabobs, 201
Zucchini Sauté, 202

Tomatoes
Cherry Tomatoes Stuffed with Crab, 6
Fettucine Verde with Tomato Sauce, 87
Gazpacho, 67
Herb-Broiled Tomatoes, 192
Marinara Sauce, 31
Pasta Salad–Stuffed Tomatoes, 50
Squash and Tomato Cassoulet, 197

Turkey
Indoor Barbecued Turkey , 119
Spicy Turkey Chili, 79
Turkey Burgers, 127
Turkey Cutlets Diane,128
Turkey Meatballs, 22
Turkey Sausage Patties, 238
Turkey with Almond Duxelles, 129

Veal
Veal Piccata with Orange Sauce, 151
Veal Romano, 152
Veal Scallopini, 153

Vegetables
Artichokes Parmesan, 183
Asparagus with Vinaigrette, 184
Broccoli with Lemon-Butter Sauce, 185
Carrots Marsala, 186
Chinese Asparagus, 187
Creamed Spinach, 188
Creole Eggplant, 189
Dill-Flavored Carrots, 190
Green Beans with Garlic and Onion, 191
Herb-Broiled Tomatoes, 192
Mushroom Cassoulets, 193
Sautéed Sweet Peppers, 194
Sherried Peppers with Bean Sprouts, 195
Snow Peas with Sesame Seeds, 196
Squash and Tomato Cassoulet, 197
Tangy Green Beans, 198
Vegetable Confetti, 199
Vegetable-Stuffed Yellow Squash, 200
Zucchini and Onion Kabobs, 201
Zucchini Sauté, 202

Other Titles Available from the American Diabetes Association

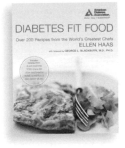

Diabetes Fit Food
By Ellen Haas

Healthy eating doesn't have to be tasteless and boring—now people with diabetes can eat the same gourmet food as everyone else! *Diabetes Fit Food* gathers amazing recipes from some of America's top celebrity chefs (including Alice Waters, Todd English, and Susan Feniger & Mary Sue Milliken) to create a one-of-a-kind cookbook that will leave you begging for more.
Order #4661-01 ✦ $16.95 US

Dr. Buynak's 1-2-3 Diabetes Diet
By Robert J. Buynak and Gregory L. Guthrie

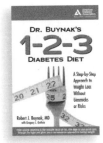

Forget fad diets. Follow Dr. Buynak's advice and get the skinny on dropping those unwanted pounds. Using three simple and sensible steps, Dr. Buynak will show you how to achieve success in healthy eating, calorie counting, exercising, eating out healthily, resisting temptations, and keeping your attitude positive. It's not always easy, but Dr. Buynak will show you that losing weight is as straightforward as 1-2-3.
Order #4881-01 ✦ $14.95 US

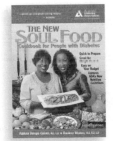

The New Soul Food Cookbook for People with Diabetes, 2nd Edition
By Fabiola Demps Gaines and Roniece Weaver

Soul food lovers rejoice! There is a cookbook just for you, and it's perfect for people with diabetes. Fabiola Gaines and Roniece Weaver have updated their popular cookbook so you can stay healthy and still enjoy great-tasting food. Most of the recipes are quick and easy, featuring just two or three steps and ingredients you'll find in any regular kitchen. So get back to basics, and bring the soul food back into your kitchen.
Order #4623-02 ✦ $14.95 US

American Diabetes Association Complete Guide to Diabetes, 4th Edition
By the American Diabetes Association

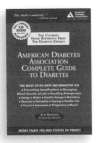

The world's largest collection of diabetes self-care tips, techniques, and tricks you can use to solve diabetes-related troubles just got bigger and better!
Order #4809-04 ✦ $29.95 US

To order these and other great American Diabetes Association titles, call **1-800-232-6733** or visit **http://store.diabetes.org**.

American Diabetes Association titles are also available in bookstores nationwide.

About the American Diabetes Association

The American Diabetes Association is the nation's leading voluntary health organization supporting diabetes research, information, and advocacy. Its mission is to prevent and cure diabetes and to improve the lives of all people affected by diabetes. The American Diabetes Association is the leading publisher of comprehensive diabetes information. Its huge library of practical and authoritative books for people with diabetes covers every aspect of self-care—cooking and nutrition, fitness, weight control, medications, complications, emotional issues, and general self-care.

To order American Diabetes Association books: Call 1-800-232-6733 or log on to *http://store.diabetes.org*

To join the American Diabetes Association: Call 1-800-806-7801 or log on to *www.diabetes.org/membership*

For more information about diabetes or ADA programs and services: Call 1-800-342-2383. E-mail: AskADA@diabetes.org or log on to *www.diabetes.org*

To locate an ADA/NCQA-Recognized Provider of quality diabetes care in your area: *www.ncqa.org/dprp*

To find an ADA-Recognized Education Program in your area: Call 1-800-342-2383. *www.diabetes.org/for-health-professionals-and-scientists/recognition/edrecognition.jsp*

To join the fight to increase funding for diabetes research, end discrimination, and improve insurance coverage: Call 1-800-342-2383. *www.diabetes.org/advocacy-and-legalresources/advocacy.jsp*

To find out how you can get involved with the programs in your community: Call 1-800-342-2383. See below for program Web addresses.

- *American Diabetes Month:* educational activities aimed at those diagnosed with diabetes—month of November. *www.diabetes.org/communityprograms-and-localevents/americandiabetesmonth.jsp*
- *American Diabetes Alert:* annual public awareness campaign to find the undiagnosed—held the fourth Tuesday in March. *www.diabetes.org/communityprograms-and-localevents/americandiabetesalert.jsp*
- *American Diabetes Association Latino Initiative:* diabetes awareness program targeted to the Latino community. *www.diabetes.org/communityprograms-and-localevents/latinos.jsp*
- *African American Program:* diabetes awareness program targeted to the African American community. *www.diabetes.org/communityprograms-and-localevents/africanamericans.jsp*
- *Awakening the Spirit: Pathways to Diabetes Prevention & Control:* diabetes awareness program targeted to the Native American community. *www.diabetes.org/communityprograms-and-localevents/nativeamericans.jsp*

To find out about an important research project regarding type 2 diabetes: *www.diabetes.org/diabetes-research/research-home.jsp*

To obtain information on making a planned gift or charitable bequest: Call 1-888-700-7029. *www.wpg.cc/stl/CDA/homepage/1,1006,509,00.html*

To make a donation or memorial contribution: Call 1-800-342-2383. *www.diabetes.org/support-the-cause/make-a-donation.jsp*

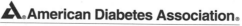